UNDERSTANDING BODYBUILDING NUTRITION & TRAINING

We learn and understand by asking questions. From the pre-schooler to the University Scholar, the fundamental way to obtain new information is by asking. Therefore, I have arranged this book in a simple, easy to understand, question and answer format.

For many, reading a book and comprehending the most important points can be difficult. With the Q & A format, I have refined longer, perhaps confusing questions, into short and focused ones. In doing so, the answers are more concise and related directly to the main topic in each question.

Finally, I suggest you read the questions and answers from beginning to end and in order, from the first page to the final page of the book since many questions build on the answers from the previous question.

*Special Thanks to photographer
Irvin Gelb
for providing all the
photos in this book.*

Copyright © 1998 by Nutramedia, Inc.
www.nutramedia.com

All rights reserved.
No portion of this book may be used or reproduced
without the author's consent.

First Printing - July 1998
Second Printing - March 1999
Third Printing - August 1999
Fourth Printing - November 1999
Fifth Printing - March 2000
Sixth Printing - January 2001
Seventh Printing - March 2003

Printed in the USA

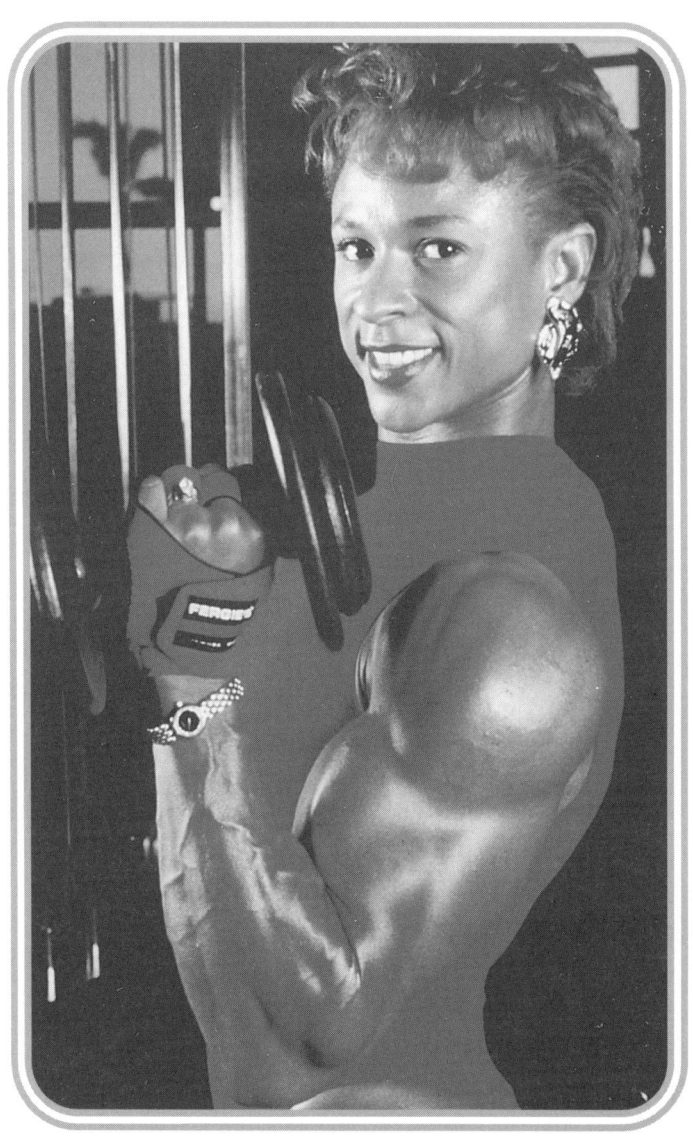

Laura Creavalle relys on sound nutrition and training to be her best.

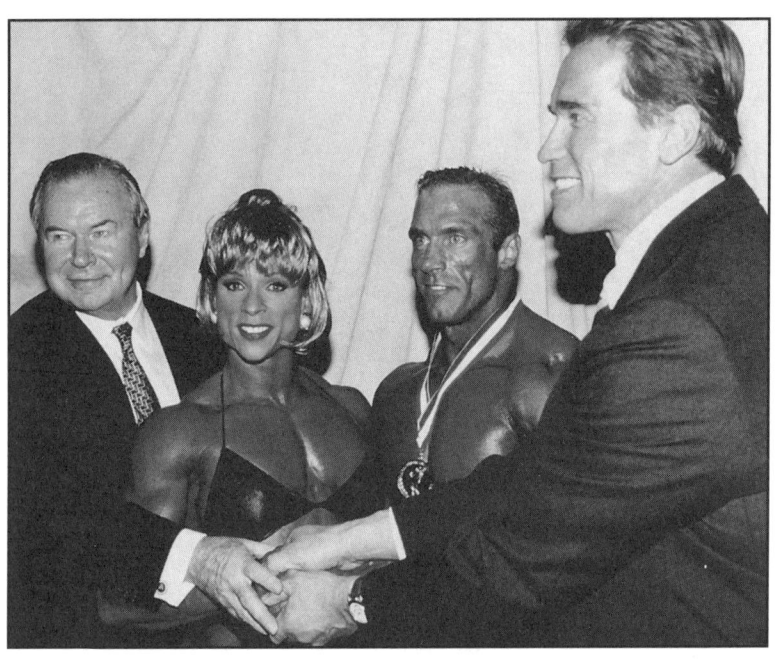

*Laura & Mike Francois enjoy the fruits of their labor.
1995 Arnold Classic Champs*

Training Questions

Q) What is the most important aspect beginning bodybuilders should focus on?
A) While it may sound extremely elementary, the **form** a beginner uses is the most important component in stimulating the muscles to grow. Correct form forces you to keep the stress on the muscle or muscle group you are targeting.

Good form prevents injuries. When a weight is just too heavy, the bodybuilder often "cheats" and resorts to poor form. Bad form shifts stress off the targeted muscle being worked and places the stress on joints; the tendons, ligaments and other muscles.

Q) What is the most important aspect of training for the advanced bodybuilder.
A) Believe it or not, form is still the most important aspect in causing muscles to grow - even for the serious athlete. As long as your form is strict, you are thoroughly working your muscle. Adding weight, using forced reps and other advanced techniques will

stimulate the muscle to grow **only** if the right form is employed.

Q) After proper form, what is the next step in causing muscle growth.
A) After mastering good form, the tension you place on the muscle is vital in causing muscle growth. The tension is also known as the "load" put on the muscle and the "load" is equal to the weights you use. Good form keeps the tension on the muscle being worked, but continual muscle growth requires you progressively, over time, increase the load. The easy way to increase the load is to add more weight to the exercises you are performing.

Q) Should females train differently than males?
A) Generally, both men and women should train the same, especially if their goal is the same; to add muscle mass. The best way to add muscle is the same whether you are a man or woman. Work with good form using a heavy weight.

Q) Should older people train differently than younger people.
A) Again, the answer is no. They should train the same; with good form and with progressively heavier weights.

The main difference between a 50 year old and a 20 year old, either male or female, is recovery time. Younger people can recover faster than older people. Therefore, a younger person can train more frequently than an older person due to superior recovery. However, they shouldn't train **differently.**

Q) I am primarily interested in increasing my strength. What is the best rep range.

A) If you wish to increase your strength, then you should train in the 3 to 5 repetition range, even doing some sets of 1 and 2 reps. The muscles adapt to low rep training **primarily** by becoming stronger. You've probably seen Olympic lifting on t.v. or maybe you know someone in your gym who is a powerlifter. Some of these athletes are tremendously strong, yet do not "look" it. They are not as "big" as they are strong. This is due to the rep range they use. Training under 6 reps allows you to become stronger, but not dramatically bigger.

Q) If I am bodybuilding, I should avoid the lower rep ranges?

A) No. It seems the best rep range for muscle growth is somewhere between 6 to 12 reps. Your Muscles adapt to the 6 to 12 rep range by becoming **primarily** bigger, **secondary** stronger. So, you will become both big and strong in by training in the 6 to 12 rep range.

One thing muscle physiologists know for sure is this; "muscles adapt to a greater tension by becoming larger" The twist is the rep range. Muscles will get stronger in the lower rep range and bigger in the 6 to 12 rep range. If your goal is to add mass, train (mostly) in the 6 to 12 rep range but on occasion, increase the poundage even further and train with even heavier weights in the 2 to 5 rep range. This will increase your strength and when you return to sets that incorporate 6 to 12 reps, you will have a "carry over" effect and be able to use greater weights and put greater tension on the muscle in the 6 to 12 rep range.

Q) How often should I use the lower rep range?
A) Try training for 2 full months in the 6 to 12 rep range. Then train exclusively in the lower rep range for 2 full weeks before returning to the 6 to 12 rep range.

Q) What's the best rep range for adding mass?
A) 6 to 12 reps for each set, but try 3 to 5 reps from time to time to increase strength.

Q) Aren't size and strength correlated?
A) Yes, size and strength are correlated **in the right rep range**-6 to 12. Therefore, you should train in the 6 to 12 rep range. Those who train exclusively in the lower rep range, 5 reps and under, will experience improvements in strength with smaller increases in muscle size.

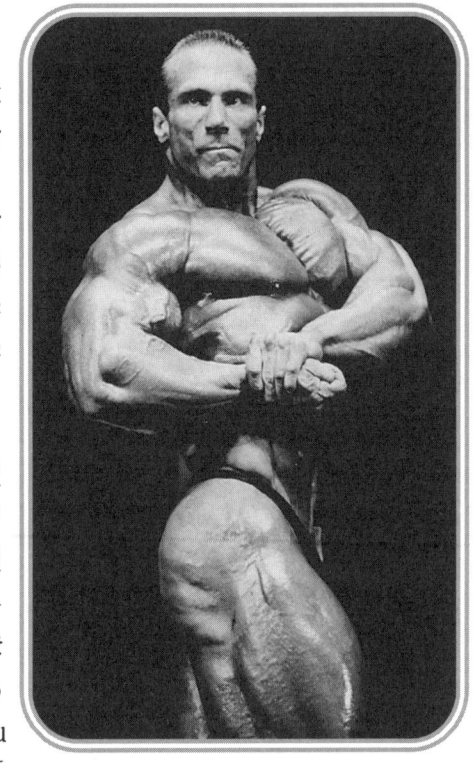

Mike built his mass with a combination of heavy weights in the 6-12 rep range and heavier weights in the 3-5 range.

Q) Describe what is meant by "explosion"
A) Explosion means pushing the weight you are lifting with great speed. The "faster" you push a weight, the more force created. In effect, when you push with speed or in an explosive fashion, you force your muscle to work "harder" and you are able to lift more weight. When you perform your reps, they should be performed with "speed" and "aggression" which allows you to handle greater poundages and, in turn, causes maximal muscle fiber recruitment.

Q) What is the best time to train?
A) Truly, the best time to train is the time that you can commit to. However, research shows that growth hormone (GH) levels in both men and women are higher in the morning. GH is also released with weight training. Therefore, training hard in the morning may exert some type of synergistic effect where you can increase GH levels even further. GH effects your progress in 2 ways. First, GH causes fat cells to break down, ultimately making you leaner. Second, GH causes muscles to "uptake" amino acids from protein foods. The muscles then incorporate these amino acids into its structure. The result is new muscle growth.

Q) How many times a week should I train?
A) This depends on 1 thing: how long you have been training. Here is a rule of thumb most everyone gets totally wrong. **The longer you have been training and the more experience you have in the gym, the less frequently you have to train!**

Beginners have really no clue as to how to do the exercises correctly and they often fear using any significant load. The result of their inexperience is this; they really aren't causing any real muscle damage or recruiting much muscle in their first 2 months of training. As you become more experienced and your pain threshold increases, your ability to use the best form possible improves, and you strive to continuously increase the tension on the muscle by increasing the load (weight). The result: the muscles truly become stressed and need more time to recover - before you train them again.

Ask any good bodybuilder. **All** of them trained more frequently the first year or two and they made good progress! To continue to make progress, they had to have pushed themselves harder and harder using heavier and heavier weights (still sticking to good form). As you train harder, you must train each body part less frequently and with a greater load (weight).

Q) I heard it takes a muscle 24 to 48 hours to recover.
A) That's inaccurate and misleading. Textbooks make that claim and here is how they came to that conclusion. Researches located on some University campus decide to address the dilemma:"How long does it take for muscles to recover" They recruit 20 college kids who are hoping to make a couple bucks during the study. The kids don't train with weights, many may have never exercised at all in their lives. All 20 perform 2 sets of bicep curls on Monday at noon. Tuesday, they return at noon to the research center. The researchers take a muscle biopsy or have the

students urinate in cups so they can check for muscle damage. Some of the students show no damage while results of others reveal the bicep muscle is still damaged. The group who show no damage gets paid and heads back to their dorm room while the researcher concludes "muscles require 24 hours to recover." Meanwhile, the other group who show muscle damage is asked to come back tomorrow (Wednesday) at noon. The students return the following day, take the tests, show they have recovered and our researches draw a second conclusion, "muscle take 48 hours to recover." The **flaw** in the statement that muscles take 24 to 48 hours to recover is simple. The body works as a unit. Had the researchers made the students train legs on Tuesday, they would have found that the stress of training on Tuesday prolonged the recovery time of the biceps. Had they taken the experiment even further and had the students train Back on Wednesday and Chest on Thursday, the results would be dramatically different. Those biceps worked on Monday may not fully recover until Friday! The body is working hard to recover from **one** workout and is being stressed over and over with **subsequent** workouts. As a rule: never train a bodypart more than once a week! When you are training ALL the bodyparts, it takes longer than 24 to 48 hours for the muscles to recover fully.

Q) How do I know I have recovered without taking biopsys or running to a University every day!?
A) If you are getting stronger, you are recovering. If you have a lot of energy during your workout **and**

during the day, you are recovering. If your muscles are growing and appear "full" in appearance, you are recovering properly.

Q) How many sets should I do for each bodypart?
A) After warm-ups, about 2 to 3 sets **for each exercise.** If you can do more, then add weight and do just 2 to 3 sets per exercise. If you are working in good form, with a heavy weight, you **can't** do more sets **without** having to reduce the weight. Reducing the weight is always a mistake.

Q) How long should I rest in between sets.
A) You should wait long enough for your heart rate to return to a near resting pulse. The goal is to cause the muscle you are working to tire on each set, to fail. Moving like a rabbit from set to set elevates the heart rate and adds stress to the cardiovascular system, making it difficult to put 100% **muscular** effort into each set. Remember, using a heavy load is important in muscle growth. If you train too fast, you can **never** handle the poundages you could if you waited longer between sets. Rest 1 minute for smaller bodyparts and 2 to 4 minutes on larger bodyparts, especially on exercises that really take a lot of effort such as bent over rows, squats, leg presses, chins, and shoulder presses. To summarize, your goal is to cause your muscles to fail while using good form, in the 6 to 12 rep range. **Muscle fatigue** is not the goal. Lots of light repetitive sets can cause fatigue without causing failure. Failure is "when you can't get any more reps because all the muscle fibers have been fully taxed"

Q) Aerobic athletes or those trying to improve their cardiovascular system monitor their heart rate for progress. As a bodybuilder, what should I monitor?

A) The **poundage** you use is the best way to measure intensity! Your only real monitoring gauge is the weights you use. If you can bench press 200 pounds for 8 reps this week and next week you can only bench press 200 pounds for 5 reps, you failed to recover fully. Either you are beginning to over train - to do too much without adequate rest **between workouts** - or you failed to support yourself nutritionally.

Q) How much weight can expect to gain in my first year of training?

A) If you do not have a problem with body fat, men can expect to add 10 pounds in their first year of training and women can add about 5 pounds. However, if you tend to be a bit soft, you can expect to gain less or even lose weight. The best way to check your progress is to have your body composition tested each week. This will tell you how much of you is fat and how much is muscle.

Q) What is meant by the term "Muscle Endurance"

A) Muscle endurance is a grey area. When you perform high reps, 15 or more, the adaptation process is neither an increase in strength nor an increase in size. Basically, you just "get better at doing it"

Try push ups for example. A 150 pound inactive male may be able to do 15 reps. Each morning he arises and adds one more push up. Six months later, he is able to do 50 push ups. The rep range is high and the adaptation is different. The weight he uses never increases and he is out of the strength rep range of 2 to 5 reps. As well, he is out of the size and strength rep range of 6 to 12 reps, so he can **not** see any real increases in muscle mass. Overall, for changes in strength or size, high reps are a waste.

Q) But I see articles featuring pro bodybuilders who use high reps.
A) Significant increases in muscle size can not be achieved with high reps. High reps will increase the blood flow to a muscle and increase the production of lactic acid, a by product in the breakdown of sugar. Although blood flow and lactic acid are mild inducers of muscle growth, large changes in mass are the result of increases in total load; the weight you use, the proper rep range and the total number of sets you do.

Q) Do high reps burn fat?
A) No. All weight training burns predominantly sugar for fuel and aerobic training burns predominantly fat as fuel. As long as you are using weights, you are burning sugar.

Q) Describe "fiber type".
A) Each of us has a genetically determined mix of special muscle fibers. Each muscle in your body is a blend of slow twitch and fast twitch muscle fibers.

Q) What does slow twitch mean?
A) Slow twitch means the muscle fiber is slow to fatigue. Slow twitch muscle fibers use fat for fuel. Marathon runners use these fibers to run. As I said, most muscle is made of a mixture of both slow and fast twitch.

Q) What are fast twitch fibers.
A) Fast twitch muscle fibers are quick to fatigue. These are the ones used for bodybuilding. In a nutshell, there

are two types of fast twitch fibers.

Q) What are the 2 kinds of fast twitch fibers?
A) The 2 types are called 2a and 2b fast twitch muscle fibers.

Q) What's the difference between the 2a and 2b fibers.
A) 2a fibers can grow by 25%. This means if you started training with a 10 inch arm, you can expect to increase the circumference by 25% or 2 inches. 2b fibers can grow by 100% in size. Therefore, a 10 inch arm has the potential to double in size to 20 inches!

Q) If I do lots of sets and reps will I be working the 2b fibers.
A) Not necessarily. In general, 2b fibers are stubborn and are worked best in the 6 to 12 rep range. Furthermore, they are very resistant to participation until you are at your "breaking point" and can barely complete the final rep of the set. When you do lots and lots of sets, you are unable to handle the heavy poundages required for muscle growth, so you rarely work the 2b fibers. Another problem with doing mega set workouts is you over train **without** working the 2b fibers. In effect, you **exhaust** yourself but fail to stimulate growth.

If mega volume was the basis for muscle growth then weight training and muscle growth would be simple (ie) "just do 40 sets for each body part and you'll look awesome."

Q) How do I train the 2b fibers?
A) First, understand that the 2a fibers always come into play when you lift weights. However, the characteristic of 2b fibers is this; **they're stubborn!** They only come into play at the very end of a set, at the last possible

moment when the set is heaviest and most difficult to accomplish. Getting at them takes a tremendous effort and maximum exertion, in good form. In addition to heavy weights, the **speed** at which you move those heavy weights influences 2b recruitment - whether you will work them properly. **Faster reps,** or trying to move a weight quickly with explosive power is a factor in causing the 2b to come into play.

Q) How can there be such a discrepancy in training. Some professional bodybuilders do 1 or 2 sets while others do 20 to 30 sets per bodypart. What gives?
A) The huge discrepancy is due to genetics. Your muscles and most everyone else's on this planet are comprised of a blend of slow twitch fibers and fast twitch fibers, both 2a and 2b. This explains why "Joe Average" could run a marathon if he wanted to put in the time required to accomplish such a task. It also explains why he can weigh a lean 215 pounds. He can build muscle with the right training and diet. However, since he has a mixture of muscle fibers, it would be impossible for him to **win** a marathon race or **win** a national bodybuilding championship.

Think about the Olympic Marathon. The US team is sponsored by Nike. The runners have the best shoes, they train under the most qualified coaches and work with top nutritionists regarding their food intake. You'd think they'd be unbeatable! What happens? They end up losing to the Ethiopian team, the Moroccan team, the Sudanese team etc. None of those teams have the Nike endorsement, the coaching etc. However, they have the overwhelming genetics that permit them to run better than anyone else. Their muscles are comprised of far greater slow twitch fibers than fast twitch fibers and slow twitch are made for endurance and cardio exercise.

Now to the bodybuilders. If one's genetic make-up dictates he has far greater fast twitch fibers than slow twitch fibers and far greater 2b fibers than 2a fibers, then **anything will work! Any type of resistance training will promote spectacular results.** Since **your** muscles are probably a mix of slow twitch and 2a and 2b fibers, your goal should be to train as intelligently as possible and work the 2b's. Too many sets will crush your ability to recover - to bounce back from each workout - and you'll fail to make big gains.

Q) What's a good indicator that I had a productive workout.
A) In this order; the weights/load used, your level of aggression, the pump. The load is your primary monitor. If you are aggressive, you are, more than likely, fully recovered, and the pump is a final indicator. It's possible to use great big weights without having a great pump, so you can't and shouldn't rely exclusively on the pump as a monitoring gauge.

Q) What If I can't use my usual poundages?
A) You are falling into an over training spiral or your diet is not supporting the stress you are putting on it.

Q) Define Overtraining.
A) Simple. Your doing too much so you are overwhelming your body. The result is no progress.

Q) How do I know If I am over training.
A) You are not making progress, your tired, going to the gym feel likes a chore, your relying on coffee and stimulants to get you through your workout, your weights are either falling or not increasing.

Q) I don't want to be a bodybuilder but I want to look muscular. What should I do? How should I train?
A) If you want to look muscular, your real goal is to shed fat and add muscle. The only way to achieve such a goal is through weight training; 6 to 12 rep sets, using heavy weights, training each body part once a week and paying special attention to your diet.

Q) What is the fuel source for weight training?
A) Sugar. This comes from carbohydrate foods.

Q) If sugar is the fuel, how can weight training possibly make me lean, and help me lose fat?
A) Weight training builds muscle. The more muscle you have, the more calories your body needs each day even at complete rest. Turns out, the human body is a fat burner at rest! While we don't burn up tremendous amounts of calories sitting around all day in front of a computer or at a desk, the fuel source for the resting body comes **overwhelmingly from fat!** Therefore, if you add muscle to your body, you need more **total calories** and **you burn more fat as fat is the predominant source of fuel at rest.**

Q) I only have time to train 2 times a week due to a crazy work schedule. Can I gain muscle training this way?
A) Not really. If you are training all the bodyparts in one training session, the bodyparts that are trained towards the end of the workout suffer because you lack the energy to train them hard enough to grow.

Q) Define Muscle Physiology.
A) Muscle Physiology is a fancy term meaning "how muscles work." It is important to grasp the ideas such as

fuel sources, rep ranges, fiber types and the like because it gives us an understanding on what really causes muscles to grow and what causes fat storage or fat loss. There are many myths and misconceptions in exercise and bodybuilding that are confusing or sound right - yet our ability to decide if the information we get in the gym is accurate is compromised by our limitations in understanding muscle physiology. If we understand the terms we can decide what is myth and what really does work.

Fortunately, with diet it is a bit easier. If you ask the leanest person in your gym "what are you doing to get so lean?" and he answers "I eat anything I want." Your likely to decide the person has a super fast metabolism and the information that works for him will not work for you. Genetically, he would be considered one with a fast metabolism. With the training the same is true. Much of the information we get may be inaccurate and handed down by those with great genetics, people with an abundance of the favorable 2b muscle fibers. Yet, it is harder to decide "Does this person really know what he is talking about?" Understanding and applying proper exercise physiology will free you from these problems.

Q) Can doing high reps make me more defined?
A) No. Definition is the result of having large muscles with as little body fat as possible. If your goal is to be ripped, train for mass and let your diet and a moderate amount of aerobic work burn off any body fat that is blurring your definition.

Q) My trainer told me 20 reps burns more fat.
A) He's wrong. All weight training burns predominantly sugar as fuel. If you want to burn fat as fuel, do aerobic

work. Even if your trainer believes high reps will stimulate fat loss, he is still giving you poor advice based on his misconceptions. If higher reps burns fat than why not do 40 reps and burn "twice as much" fat.

Q) What are supersets?
A) A Superset is an advanced technique used by bodybuilders to work the muscle harder. A superset describes performing one set immediately after another, with no or very little rest in between. I don't think they are particularly effective because when you combine two sets, the total reps will surpass 12, so you are working in the higher rep range or **endurance range.** However, you can modify your supersets and perform one set immediately after another if the total reps in the two sets combined do not surpass 12. For example, you can perform shoulder presses for 6 heavy reps then move onto (immediately with no rest) dumbbell side laterals and perform another 6 reps. This allows you to work the 2b fibers - you work as heavy as possible employing the 6 to 12 rep range.

Q) What are strip sets?
A) Stip sets are another advanced technique. Pick a heavy enough weight on any exercise that will allow you to complete (only) 4 or five reps. Immediately, take some weight off the bar or pick a lighter pair of dumbbells and perform just 2 or 3 reps. In total you have completed 6 to 8 reps with the heaviest weight possible.

Q) What is Rest-Pause?
A) This is another advanced training technique. Again, pick a heavy weight that will allow you to complete (only) 6 reps. When you are exhausted on the last rep,

rack the weight, and rest for 20 seconds. After 20 seconds, complete 2 more reps.

Q) What about Periodization.
A) Periodization may look good on paper, but in the real world, at the gyms throughout the country, nobody really uses it because it doesn't really work. Apparently, rotating heavy and light workouts will yield more progress than training hard and "all-out" all year long. I disagree completely. First, the studies are flawed. They combine 2 groups of people and show those who "cycle" their workouts make "equal or better" progress

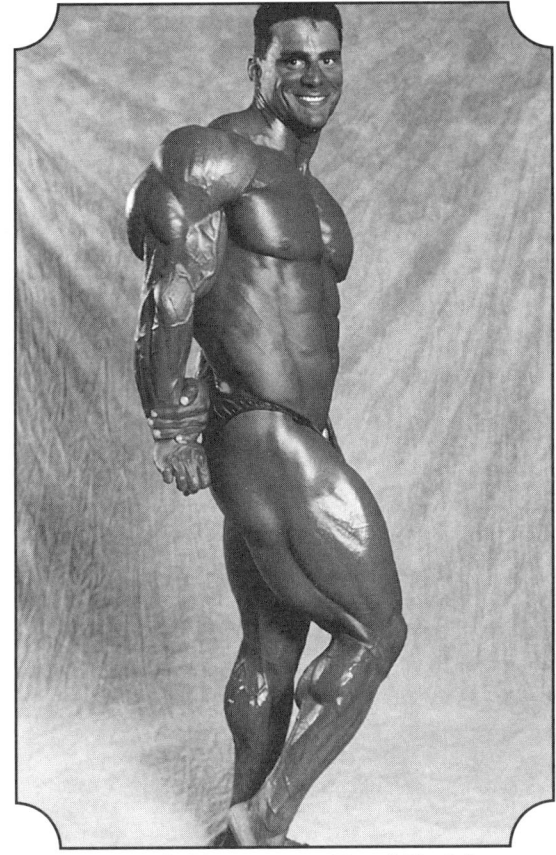

National Champion Paul DeMayo.

than those who don't cycle their workouts. A real study would compare how much progress the entire group made using periodization methods **then** find out how much progress they made using regular training methods. Finally, I think it is wiser to train all-out at every workout and take enough days off from training to allow for full recuperation and muscle growth.

Q) How important is rep speed in muscle growth.
A) Rep speed also plays a strong role in stimulating 2b muscle fibers as the speed of the contraction, movement or activity activates the nerves that are responsible for signaling the 2b fibers to "contract". Take a look at sprinters. They will get some muscle development simply as the result of their ***explosive*** super intense burst of speed. So, for optimal 2b recruitment use heavy weights **and** try to move the weight "quickly" while doing the reps. Of course, don't neglect good form as sloppy form removes the tension from the targeted muscle group.

Q) Should I do fast reps on the negative part of the reps?
A) Let's make sense of it. I already explained that good form keeps the tension on a muscle. Once you have mastered the right form, increasing your load (weight used) has the greatest impact on muscle

growth. I also explained that, for muscle growth, the ideal rep range is 6 to 12 per set. To work the muscle even harder and to recruit more of those stubborn 2b fibers, you can lower the weight at a slower pace. Under normal workout conditions, you probably take 1 to 1.5 seconds to lower a weight.

On the last rep of a set, try taking 2 to 3 seconds to lower the weight. While the load has not changed, you have put more total stress on the muscle causing more muscle growth.

Q) So I can vary my workouts by changing the speed at which I do my reps.
A) Yes. However, still try to use as heavy as a weight as possible and push fast and aggressively during the positive part of the rep as speed with a heavy weight influence 2b growth.

Q) Define "positive" and "negative"
A) "Positive" is the action the muscle take when **doing** each exercise. In the 6 to 12 rep range, the more weight you handle, the **more** muscle fibers come into play. In essence the weight you handle and speed at which you move that weight in the positive direction **influence how many total muscle fibers you recruit** or include.

The "Negative" is the part of the rep where you "resist" the weight. All muscles are stronger during the negative part of the rep versus the "positive" part of the rep. Lowering the weight on the "negative" on the final rep with more control allows you to stress the muscles fibers further. However, to get **more total fibers involved,** you have to use a heavier weight on the "positive".

Q) Isn't variation the "key" to muscle growth?
A) Not really. Putting more stress on the muscle is the most important factor in muscle growth. (in regards to training) Many are under the misconception that changing their workouts around all the time is good for growth.

Q) I thought it was good for muscle growth.
A) It **may** be, **but** most start varying their workouts far too early in their training life. It is best to stick with the "basic" core exercises. Build your strength and size from those. When you start to see a slow down in progress, you can vary the workouts. Before switching exercises and angles, use advanced techniques on the very same exercises you have been doing in order to work the muscle harder.

Q) What are the techniques to work the muscle harder?
A) Control the speed on the negative part of the exercises (on the final rep, the one that is causing muscular failure), use an explosive motion on the positive, perform strip sets, rest pause and modified super sets.

Q) What are the basic core exercises?
A) The basic core are the exercises for large muscle groups that allow you to push the maximum amount of weight on that bodypart. It is much easier to distinguish which are the core or basic exercises on large bodyparts like chest, shoulders, legs and back. For example, the bench press is a core exercise for the chest. Anyone can bench press more than they can incline bench press and the same person can handle a greater load on incline bench presses than on dumbbell flies.

Q) Why is that?
A) Good question! The reason the bench press is **the** core exercise for the chest is because it works the best! It works the best for this reason; you can use the most amount of weight, more so than on other chest exercises. The more weight you can handle, the greater the stress on the **entire** bodypart. The reason you can use so little weight on flies is because it does not recruit all the muscle fibers in the chest area.

Q) So bench presses are best for chest development because I can use a lot of weight which recruits all the fibers in the chest?
A) Exactly!

Q) But I was told inclines work the upper chest more than flat bench presses.
A) That's sort of a myth. Try this out. Go to the gym and do 30 sets of bench press. No doubt you will be excruciatingly sore the next day in every part of your chest including the "upper pecs." If flat benches didn't recruit the upper pecs, as many believe, then you shouldn't be sore in the upper pec region on the following day.

Q) What does inclines do?
A) They shift the stress from the chest to the upper chest and front delts. If you fail on the incline, your chest muscles and more of the shoulder region come into play together.

Q) What are the core exercises for the other bodyparts.
A) Squats are best for legs, though there is not a lot of difference between squats and leg presses. Shoulder presses over the head with a bar or dumbbell shoulder

presses are the number one exercise for total shoulder development and bent over rows and chins are great for back development.

Q) What about biceps and triceps?
A) Arms are a bit different. First, they are trained twice as often as other bodyparts as biceps come into play while working back and triceps receive a lot of stress by training chest and shoulders.

The point is arms can easily get too much work and, subsequently, fail to grow. The other interesting aspect regarding arms is that most exercises are variations of each other. No one bicep or tricep exercise seems to be radically better than another. For example dumbbell curls versus machine curls. Both are pretty equal. Both cause you to simply bend at the elbow, causing the bicep to contract. Since the elbow joint is a fairly simple joint, the exercises do not need to be complex.

Q) How can I track my progress?
A) This may be the best question of all. If you are serious about measuring your progress, you must keep a training (and diet) log, take photos from time to time, usually once a month, and keep a log of your body composition changes. In your training log should record the exercises you do, the weights used and the number of sets and reps. Repeat the same workouts over and over. DO NOT change. Your log, over time should tell you this; that your workouts are working-you are making progress by increasing muscle mass or your log will show you are making very little progress. If you do make progress, DO NOT CHANGE A THING in your training. Never mess with a successful formula. At best,

you can "fine tune" your training in an attempt to accelerate progress. You can add a strip set, add a couple or forced reps, etc, but do not deviate from a working/successful formula. If you are not making progress, then you are clearly training wrong and must evaluate your training (and diet) log to see where you may have gone wrong.

One thing I can tell you for sure; unless you have outstanding genetics for building muscle, you won't be able to "wing it" and make serious progress in building your body unless you keep clear records

Q) Should I be sore after training?
A) In general, sore muscle are a good indicator you had a productive workout. However, you should not be extremely sore. That's an indicator you probably worked the muscle too hard or with too many sets. If you are sore for more than two full days after training a muscle, you may probably over worked that area.

Q) Should I train fast to increase the intensity of my workouts?
A) Training fast, waiting a very brief time in between workouts, is absurd! Imagine Carl Lewis running a 100 meter sprint and walking back to the staring blocks to repeat the 100 meter run. He'd be dead tired! Weight training is the **opposite** of aerobic training. In aerobics, like distance running, the movement is long, slow and **continuous.** Anaerobic sports like sprinting and weight training require huge bursts of energy. The actual movement is rapid and quick. Think about the 100 meters or a 10 rep heavy set. Either takes less than 12 seconds but the athlete is "beat" tired after the sprint or

after the set. Replenishing his energy requires recovery and recovery requires **time.** So, moving fast between sets is a way to **decrease** your intensity!

Remember, the aerobic athlete likes to track and measure his "intensity." He does this by recording his heart rate. We bodybuilders record our intensity **by the poundage we use.** Train slower, rest adequately between sets, and the weights you can handle will increase and, in time, your mass will also increase.

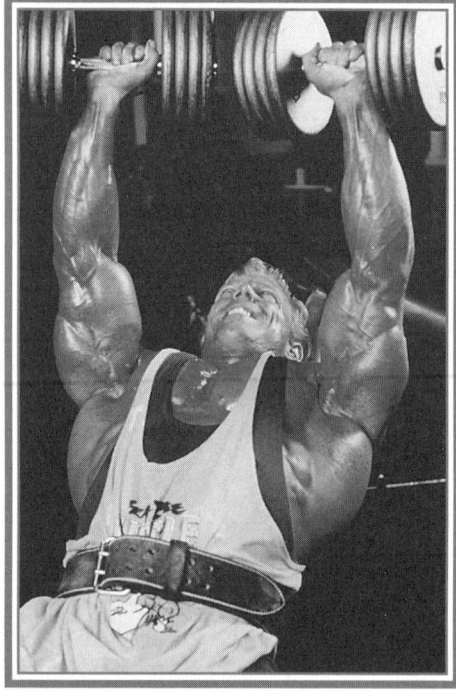

Dave Fischer rests long enough between sets to perform with maximal poundages.

Q) What about body fat. Should I keep track of it?
A) Absolutely. If your **bodyweight** is increasing, you know your getting more "massive." However, most will add a combination of mass made of both lean body weight or muscle and body fat.

Q) What device should I use to measure my fat?
A) Most fat measuring devices are not very accurate. However, all of them are consistent in measuring a **change** in body fat. You may (in reality) be 10% body fat, but the device measures you as 8%. If you lose 5 pounds of fat your percentage of fat will go down (equally) on **both** an accurate device and inaccurate device. One device may now record you as 8% and the other 6%. Both devices record you as falling the same amount; 2%. In summary, body fat measuring devices may not be "dead on" accurate, though they are accurate in measuring the change in fat levels.

Q) Should I look to gain 100% pure muscle with no body fat?
A) That would be ideal, but that's not how it works in the real world. If you weigh 170 pounds and, over time, gain 10 pounds, your total weight increased by 10 pounds. **As long as you gain more muscle than fat,** your headed in the right direction.

Q) What do you mean by headed in the right direction?
A) If you gained 6 pounds of muscle and 4 pounds of fat, you have become leaner! Obviously, if you went from 170 to 180 pounds and gained more fat than muscle, your headed in the wrong direction - your getting fatter. The ideal is to add 2 to 3 pounds of muscle for each pound of fat. Therefore if you gained 9 total pounds on the scale, your muscle should increase by 6 pounds and your fat by 3 pounds (maximum).

The net effect is a very positive change in body composition.

Q) How much sleep does a bodybuilder need each night?
A) I know all the best bodybuilders love to sleep at least 8 hours a night with a 1 to 2 hour nap in the afternoon. That's what they do because it works. I never have been able to grow unless I sleep 9 hours a night.

Q) Is it too late to start weight training. I'm a fifty year old woman and am out of shape
A) It is a cliche, but it is never too late. A friend of mine I trained never worked out in any way shape or form until he was 61 but by the time he reached 65, he became a competitive bodybuilder! While it is impossible for a 60 year old to make the progress of a 20 year old, both the 60 and 20 year old can radically re-shape their physiques.

Q) What is the best training split to add mass?
A) In general, most people who are seeking mass can not recover adequately from more than 2 consecutive workouts in a row. For this reason, I like the the 2 day on 1 day rest split. A common way to split the bodyparts are as follows. Day 1 train chest and shoulders. Day 2 train legs. Rest on day 3. Come back and train Back on day 4 and arms on day 5. Rest again on day six, then repeat the full cycle.

Q) Why do others train on different splits than the one you suggest?
A) Think about this; it's not the total number of workouts in a year that determine your success in adding muscle. It's the total number of **productive** workouts that determine your success in adding muscle mass.

Therefore, people split up their workouts to **maximize recovery.** Some recover slower than others and some recover faster than others. I suggest you pick the workout schedule that allows for complete recovery.

Q) How do I know If I have recovered completely?
A) Recovered muscles are strong muscles. If you are getting stronger or feel good in the gym, you are recovering. If your poundages are falling or have stagnated, you are not recovered fully.

Q) How do I make sure I recover fully?
A) The only way to maximize recovery is through proper eating and rest. If your not fully recovered you must take an extra day off from your training or you can change your split so you are training each body part less frequently.

Q) How many sets per bodypart should I do for each body part?

A) That is a good and tough question to answer. First realize the more experience you have, the harder you can push yourself in the gym. Second, the more sets you do is not the "magic bullet" in regards to muscle stimulation and muscle growth.

If **total volume** was the key to muscle growth, the answer to your question would be easy. I'd suggest 20 to 30 sets a bodypart. However, since volume is not the answer, we should look at the other end of the spectrum. Mike Mentzer claims 1 set is best for muscle growth. While he is correct in his accessment that most bodybuilders over train by doing too many sets, he is ignorant in his misconception that one set is enough for everyone to cause optimal muscle growth.

The goal with your training is to recruit those stubborn 2 b muscle fibers as they have they greatest potential for muscle growth. If I told you to go into the gym and perform 25 sets for chest, you would surely have to "pace" yourself and not give 100% into each and every set. If you did put 100% effort into each and every set, you would not make it to set number 25. However, if I told you to perform just one set for your total chest workout, you would 1) think it impossible to grow on just one set and 2) you'd put every ounce of effort and every muscle fiber into working that one set to total muscle failure.

With several sets you pace yourself and rarely work the 2b fibers and with one set you work the 2b fibers. The question becomes "Do the 2b fibers need just one set?" Based on anecdotal evidence, muscles require between 4 to 12 all out sets for each bodypart to fully recruit the 2b fibers and promote optimal muscle growth.

The other reason 1 set or excessive sets will not cause muscle growth is because weight training stimulates the release of hormones that support muscle growth. With 1 set, we see a minute spike in these hormones and with excessive sets, we see a small spike accompanied with a large spike is stress hormones that inhibit muscle growth.

Q) How about scientific evidence. How many sets should I do?

A) No "scientific" evidence actually exists to prescribe the **exact** number of sets required for optimal muscle growth. However, we can rely on thousands of bodybuilders who have radically transformed their physiques through years of training and record keeping. While I haven't interviewed thousands myself, I know that the norm seems to be between 4 and 12 **total** sets for each bodypart.

Q) That's still a big discrepancy. Which bodyparts requires closer to 12?
A) Smaller bodyparts like calves and biceps and triceps requires 4 to 8 sets. You could pick 2 exercises and perform 2 to 4 sets per exercise.

Larger muscles like back, legs, shoulders and chest require between 8 and 12 total sets. In general, larger bodyparts can withstand more sets than smaller ones.

Q) How do I know if my chest requires 8 or 12 sets?
A) The number of sets to choose depends on 3 factors; strength, energy levels and your recovery ability. When your strength fails, you should move onto another exercise. For example, you are performing the bench press with 250 pounds for 8 reps and complete 2 sets. On the third set, you can barely perform 5 reps, your chest has been fully worked as your muscles don't have the ability to continue using an appropriate load. It is best to move onto your next exercise. If you continue with the bench press, the load you can handle will fall with each successive set.

If your energy is low, you probably need more days off from training and if the poundage you use on the chest exercise is lower than a previous exercise, your body, especially the muscles you are working, have not recovered.

Q) What happens if I work my chest when I am tired or when I lack strength?
A) Training when you are tired is a waste of time. Tired muscles are under-recovered muscles and under-recovered muscles can not grow even if you maintain a great diet. Weak muscles are also an indicator that you are over training or not taking enough rest days to facilitate total recovery. Muscles can not grow unless they have had ample time and proper nutrition to support recovery.

Q) What about warm ups?
A) The goal of warm up sets is to get blood into the muscles being worked to prevent injury

Q) How heavy should the warm up set be?
A) Light! Most beginners and intermediates warm up with a weight that is just too heavy. This prevents them from having the ability to push **maximum** loads. Use a very light weight for your warm up set. Perform 2 or 3 warm up sets if you wish. Remember; the warm up set is a way to get blood into the area so you can quickly move to a heavier weight without getting hurt. Warm up sets should never be taxing to your energy and strength.

Remember, using a maximum load with good form in the 6 to 12 rep range is the fastest and most effective way to recruit the 2b muscle fibers - the ones that have the greatest potential for growth.

Q) After I have performed 1 to 3 easy and light warm up sets, should I jump up to the heaviest weight I can handle on each exercise?

A) Technically, the answer is yes. After getting blood into the muscles, you should put on the heaviest weight possible and work that set to failure in the 6 to 12 rep range. Unfortunately, this could result in injury. Therefore, you must **pyramid** up to your heaviest possible weight.

Q) What do you mean by pyramid?

A) Pyramid means you should add weight gradually. The catch-22 with pyramiding is that **any set other than a maximum effort set is a waste of time** as sub maximal effort sets do not require all the muscle fibers in each muscle to come into play. Therefore, the sets between your warm ups and maximal set should be **limited** in reps to conserve your energy.

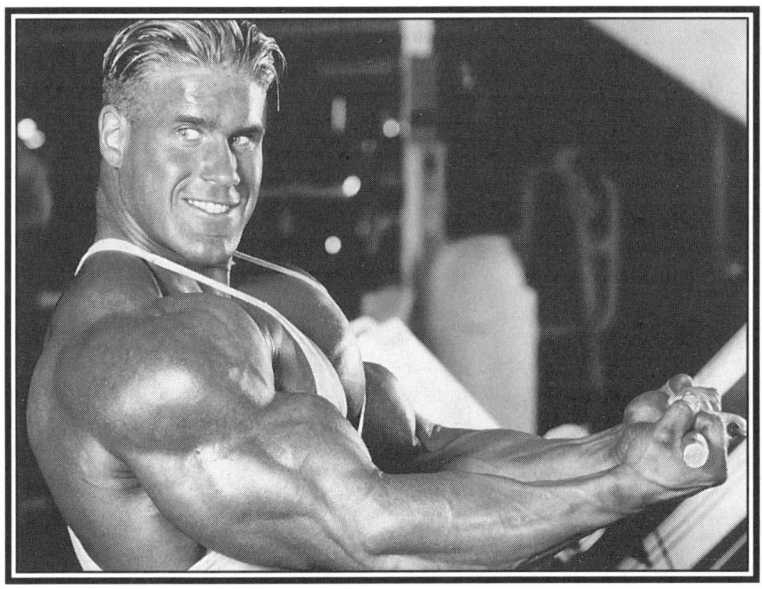

Jay uses heavy-strict form on all his exercises.

Q) Can you give me an example?
A) If you can bench press 315 pounds for 8 reps, we know it takes 315 pounds to cause your muscles to fail. When you fail and can not do anymore reps, all the muscle fibers in the chest have been recruited and worked. Your warm up should be very light. Perhaps 135 pounds for 2 easy sets of 10 reps. **Technically,** after performing your warm ups, you should jump up to 315 pounds and blast your chest while you are full of energy and strength. However, to prevent injury, you will have to pyramid and do some intermediary sets before you load 315 onto the bar. Therefore, you can do a set with 190 and another with 245 pounds. However, you should not waste energy doing sets of 6 to 12 reps with these lighter weights. Instead, perform 2 or 3 reps. Then bring the weight up to 315 pounds and do your ***first real*** set with the heavy weight. Avoiding too much unnecessary work between your warm up set and your first real set is the key to staying fresh during your workout which enables you to push maximum weights.

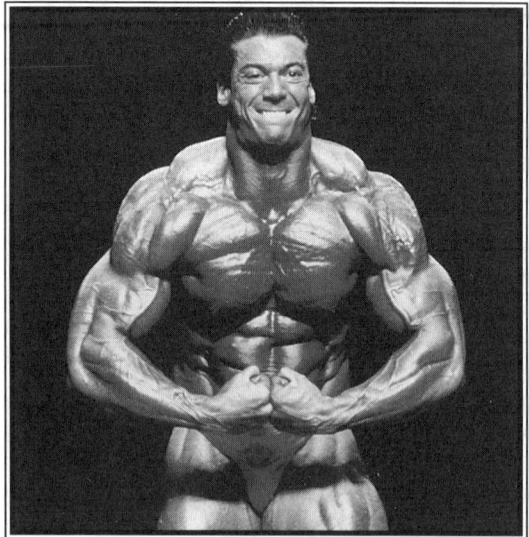

Gerard Dente's physique says "Power!"

Q) After performing my first exercise, should I move onto the second and warm up again?
A) No! After performing your first exercise, it is a waste of energy and effort to "re-warm-up."

Q) What should I do on my second exercise?
A) You should immediately put on the heaviest weight possible and work the bodypart to failure in the 6 to 12 rep range.

Q) Should I count my warm up sets and pyramid sets when tallying the total number of sets I need for each bodypart?
A) No. Each bodypart requires about 4 to 12 total sets. Only count your maximal-effort sets in this total. Do not count warm ups and the sets in between warm ups. Only include your heavy - to failure sets in your total set tally.

Q) Is there truth to the "No Pain No Gain" slogan?
A) Yes. Success does not come easy. Building muscle mass requires the lifter to stimulate the maximum amount of muscle fibers in a muscle. Muscle stimulation is accomplished by placing a lot of stress on the muscles. The stress is proportional to the weights/poundages you use and the total number of sets. Stressing the muscles causes small micro tears and these tears indicate the muscles have been thoroughly worked.

So, heavy weights recruit the maximum amount of muscle fibers in each muscle and cause small tears in the muscles which indicate the muscles have been thoroughly worked.

Q) How sore should I be after training?
A) You should be sore after training but not excessively sore. If you train chest on Monday and are scheduled to work the chest again on Sunday, then you are "too sore" In general, a muscle should be sore from 1 to 4 days after training. Therefore, if you train chest on Monday it is "ok" for it to feel sore or fatigued on Tuesday (day 1) and even up to Friday, 4 days later.

Q) What if I am still sore 5 days after training a bodypart.
A) If you are still sore then you either worked that muscle with too much volume - you did too many total sets and it is taking a very long time to recover or your nutritional intake can not support muscle recovery.

Q) What if I train a body part while it is still sore?
A) You are making a terrible mistake. Muscles can not grow unless they have totally recovered and repaired themselves from the previous training session.

Q) Is it ok to train a muscle if it is only slightly sore?
A) No! When a muscle is even slightly sore, it has failed to rebuild itself from the previous training session. If you train it in an under recovered state, you accelerate catabolism!

Q) What do you mean by catabolism?
A) Catabolism means "muscle wasting." When you train a muscle and cause slight muscle tears, the muscles are literally "torn down" While tearing down muscle does not sound like a good idea, it is a must if

you aspire to add lots of muscle mass because the body responds by releasing hormones and enzymes that fight the "tear down" state. These hormones and enzymes promote an anabolic state or "building state" In essence tearing down the muscles via hard workouts sets in motion a response by the body to rebuild the muscles. If you eat the right diet and don't overtrain and do too much work in each training session, the body not only repairs itself and builds the muscles back to their previous size, but to a bigger and larger size.

Q) What are the hormones you talked about?
A) When you train too long or when you train a sore muscle, the body releases cortisol, a stress hormone that can tear down muscle tissue. However, if you train very hard, but avoid long workouts and never train when you are too tired or sore, the body (in conjunction with a good diet) will release hormones such as insulin, growth hormone and testosterone that will support muscle growth.

Q) So, I should not train when I am sore?
A) Exactly. You should avoid overtraining. Each individual must balance their training with rest. Some people can recover faster than others. The training routines you see in bodybuilding magazines may not always be applicable to you as some bodybuilders you read about may be using drugs to speed up and enhance muscle recovery and others are very gifted in that they can recover faster than the average person.

Q) Are there other signs I should look for besides being overly sore, that could impede my muscle growth?
A) Losses in strength are associated with overtraining, a lack in "muscle pump", the need for a strong cup of coffee before training, and a lack of aggression in the gym are signs you are overtraining.

Q) What is the difference between concentric and eccentric?
A) Concentric is the word to describe the "shortening" of a muscle while eccentric describes its "lengthening." A muscle shortens when you "do" the exercise. This is also referred to as muscle "contraction." For example, when doing curls for the biceps, the bicep muscle contracts and shortens while you bring the weight up towards the body and it lengthens when you lower the weight. Likewise, when you are squatting for leg development, the muscles shorten and contract when you come "out of the hole," when you are pushing the weight up. The muscles of the legs lengthen when you descend with the weight on your back.

Q) What is more important, the concentric or eccentric part of the rep?
A) They are equally important. However, your muscles are stronger during the eccentric portion. Haven't you noticed you may fail doing a bench press. You can't "get the weight up" but can resist and control the weight on the way down. Basically, when you fail during a set and can no longer complete any more reps, you have only failed concentrically, not eccentrically!

An advanced technique to really overload and

stimulate a muscle is to incorporate negatives into your program.

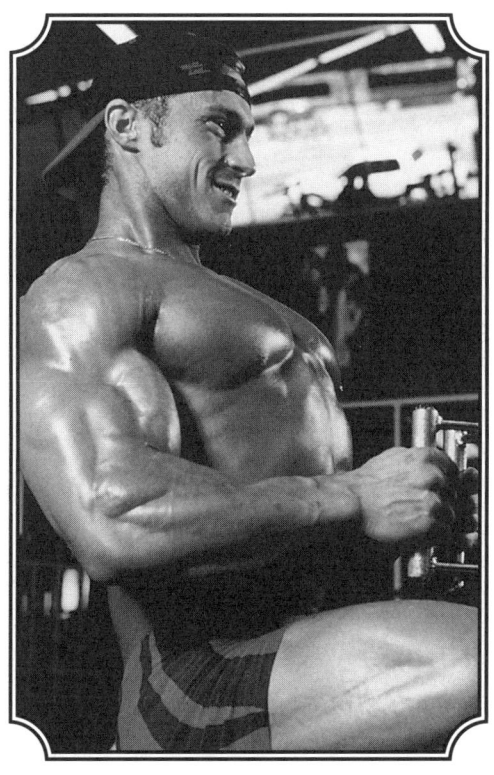

Remi resists with all his might during the last rep of his set.

Q) What are negatives?

A) Negatives allow you to ***fully*** overload and exhaust every muscle fiber in the muscle you are training. When you get to the point where you can not complete any more reps, have your partner help you do 1 or two more reps. Have him lift the weight for you during the concentric portion and you should control the weight during the eccentric portion of the rep. Do this for 2 reps maximum, at the end of a set.

Q) What is the benefit?

A) You benefit in two ways. First, you are failing both concentrically and eccentrically. Most bodybuilders only fail concentrically so they aren't truly fully taxing their muscles during each set. The other benefit involves muscle re-growth or muscle re-modeling. When you stress a muscle, growth factors are released from within the muscle tissue to set up and jump start the recovery and rebuilding process. The vast majority of these growth factors are stimulated during the eccentric portion of the reps, not during the concentric portion.

Q) So for a muscle to grow, you should tax it concentrically and eccentrically.
A) Exactly.

Q) So the eccentric is more important for muscle growth?
A) They are both important. For a muscle to grow, it must contract and lengthen, also referred to as shortening and lengthening. The load you add to the shortening and lengthening dictates the amount of stress you put on the muscles. The more stress, the better. An advanced way to get the most out of each set is to exhaust the muscle in the 6 to 12 rep range during the concentric and eccentric portions of the reps.

Q) Ok, so far I understand the stuff you have been saying. Just give me the perfect workout.
A) Unfortunately, there is no one perfect workout that everyone can use to pack on mass.

Q) Why?
A) People are different! Some recover very fast and should train more frequently. Others require more rest between workouts to allow their muscles to fully recover. As a group, bodybuilders should follow some basic principles; train heavy, eat right, use the basic

exercises, use good form, take your sets to failure, avoid overtraining, etc..

Q) Can you suggest a training split.
A) Those who wish to gain significant amounts of muscle mass often end up overtraining. To maximize your recovery ability and growth, you must rest to allow the body to fully recover. Fully recovered muscles are strong muscles and strong muscles are big muscles. The best training split limits the workouts to no more than two consecutive days. For example, if you train on Monday and Tuesday, you should rest on Wednesday before training again on Thursday and Friday. Here is an easy split that limits your training to no more than two days in a row. Day 1 train back and biceps, Day 2 train chest and abs, rest on Day 3, return to the gym and train legs and calves on Day 4, train shoulders and triceps on Day 5 and rest again on Day 6. Then repeat this cycle.

Q) What about training four days in a row followed by one day of rest?
A) While this split could work, it is flawed in that, over time, your workout intensity decreases as the week progresses. For example, by the 3rd or 4th cycle into the split, you are still having a great training session on the first day which follows your day off. However, by the 3rd day, your ability to "push" yourself in the gym falls and on the fourth day, the day before your rest day, you lack the power and energy to work hard and stimulate the muscles.

Q) What are the best exercises for each bodypart?

A) The ones that allow you to move the greatest amount of weight.

Q) Give me an example
A) Leg presses and squats are the best exercises for quads. You can develop great quadraceps, and pretty good hamstrings too, from either of these two exercises. You can not build great legs from leg extensions! Squats are better than extensions because they recruit more muscle fibers. Squats are also superior because you can handle more weight. The more weight you can handle, the more muscle fibers in the targeted area (muscle) come into play.

Bench presses are the best exercise for the chest because you can handle more weight on this exercise than any other chest exercise. When you fail with a weight, the entire chest area comes into play. ALL the muscle fibers are recruited with heavy weights. They (the fibers) come into play and contract in order to "help out" and allow you to complete the rep(s).

Q) Many beginners avoid squats and presses?
A) Unfortunately, they are training incorrectly if they are avoiding the very best exercise for legs. Many believe they can do leg extensions, lunges, hacks, etc and develop great legs. Great legs come through hard work; stay with squats and presses primarily!

Q) I'm, a woman and do not want to build I just want to tone. How should I lift?
A) There is no such word in muscle physiology as "tone." There are words like body fat, muscle, hypertrophy (muscle growth) and atrophy (muscle

shrinkage). No where, will you find the word "tone." Sometimes, women are under the impression that they will start lifting weights and blow up with an overabundance of muscle and look like a muscular man. IT CAN NOT AND WILL NOT HAPPEN! When a woman refers to "toning" she hopes to lose fat and "replace" her jiggles with firm muscle. Physiologically speaking, she must shed body fat and increase her muscle mass. Unfortunately, the word "mass" tends to scare her so she embarks on a low calorie diet coupled with the wrong weight training program. Most of her training incorporates very light weights, very high reps, and exercises that do not recruit the most amount of muscle fibers. As a result, she never adds any muscle mass. Hoping to become "toned" she loses some fat via the diet but never really "replaces" her jiggles with any muscle. Muscle is the only thing that makes someone look firm and hard. After all, it is muscle that exerts the greatest effect on your metabolism allowing you to burn more fuel, more total calories and more total fat each day even at rest. Adding muscle through heavy weight training combined with the right diet will yield a lean body.

Q) If I want to lose fat should I concentrate on weight training or aerobic training?
A) If you want to change your body composition, you should concentrate primarily on weight training and secondary on aerobic work.

Q) Define body composition.
A) Body composition is also referred to as "percent body fat" The term percent body fat is misleading. When a

person joins a gym, many have their body fat measured. Whether the test be a skin caliper, electro-impedance, or any other type of test, all measure two things 1) how much fat you have and 2) how much muscle you have.

The problem with the test can be found in its name. Because it is referred to as a percent **body fat** test, those who take the test typically wish to "improve" their results. They do so by attempting to lower the amount of fat they carry. If a person is 18% fat he wants to lower his fat to 14% The person who is 12% tries to lower his number to 8% and the person who is 8% wants to lower his percent fat measurement to 5%.

The typical approach to lose the fat is a strict diet or aerobic exercise or a combination of a diet and aerobics. While diets and aerobics work to shed and lower body fat, the smarter choice is to **increase muscle mass!** Remember, the "percent body fat test" is a ratio test. It tells you how much fat you are carrying **and** it tells you how much muscle mass you have. Altering your "percentage" can be achieved by losing fat **or** by adding muscle.

If you are very fat (higher than 30% for women and 20% for men) you should concentrate on aerobics to lose fat and lower your fat stores. Women between 20 and 30% fat should split their time between aerobics to lose fat and weight training to increase muscle. Men between 15 and 20% fat should also split their training time and allot half their time to aerobics to shed fat and the other half to weight training to add muscle mass.

Women who are less than 20% should spend the majority of time trying to add muscle mass to improve their ratio of fat to muscle. Men who are less than 15% should also spend the majority of time adding muscle mass through weight training to alter their composition.

MEN (CATEGORIES 1,2,3)

CATEGORY	PERCENT FAT	TYPE OF EXERCISE
1	more than 20%	aerobics
2	15% to 20%	weights and aerobics
3	less than 15%	spend more time on weights, less on cardio

WOMEN (CATEGORIES 1,2,3)

CATEGORY	PERCENT FAT	TYPE OF EXERCISE
1	more than 30%	aerobics
2	20% to 30%	weights and aerobics
3	less than 20%	spend more time on weights, less on aerobics

THE FOLLOWING 14 QUESTIONS PERTAIN TO THOSE INDIVIDUALS WHO FALL INTO CATEGORY 1.

Q) Can't I lower my body fat to as low level as I want with cardio?
A) Cardio exercise is primarily good for heavy people. Cardio exercise burns fat as fuel. Heavy individuals should start with cardio exercise first, before embarking on weight training.

Q) Why should the obese start with aerobics?
A) A lean person uses fat as fuel at rest. When I sit, I burn very few calories each hour, perhaps 80 to 90.

However, 2/3 of these 80 calories comes from fat and 1/3 comes from sugar. The fat my body burns at rest comes from dietary fat I may have eaten or from stored body fat. The sugar comes from what is found in the blood as "blood sugar" or from stored sugar in the muscle called muscle glycogen.

Fat people are the exact opposite. At rest, **they burn a disproportionate amount of sugar** and radically less fat. The result is twofold. First, they rarely tap into their fat stores. Second, they burn more sugar. Much of this sugar comes from their blood stream. When some of this sugar is burned up, blood sugar levels fall which, in turn, stimulates the appetite. A person with a low blood sugar level craves more sugar!

Q) How does aerobics help?
A) Aerobics increase the enzymes in the body that burn fat. Fat people have less of these enzymes. Starting with aerobics is the best choice for the obese because aerobics will build up fat burning enzymes. In time, as they lose fat by burning more calories via exercise, they will burn more fat at rest and less sugar.

Q) Why don't you suggest any weight training for the obese?
A) Weight training uses sugar as fuel. This sugar comes from the carbohydrate foods a person eats. However, the obese burn a lot of sugar at rest. When they lift weights, they also, like any lean person, use sugar as fuel.

The problem is the obese are "over using" sugar

from the blood stream during training. Their blood sugar levels drop off and they feel dizzy and light headed.

Q) Why do they feel light headed and dizzy?
A) The brain can only use sugar as fuel (and ketones). When a fat person, who already uses a lot of sugar as fuel, lifts weights, he uses up valuable sugar from the blood, thereby depriving the brain of fuel.

Q) But lean people use up lots of sugar too. How come the lean individual does not fell dizzy?
A) Lean people do not become dizzy because they "by pass" using up blood sugar as fuel. Lean people use **stored** sugar as fuel, called glycogen. At rest, the lean individual burns more fat than sugar. When he starts to burn sugar during weight training the body uses the sugar that is stored in the muscle (as muscle glycogen). **Lean people are good sugar storers.** When they eat sugar from carbohydrates, a lot is stored as glycogen - to be used later during weight training.

The obese are a different kind of sugar storer. The **obese tend to store sugar as body fat - not as muscle glycogen.** Therefore, they are continually storing fat from carbohydrate foods and continually lack sufficient muscle glycogen stores to serve as a fuel tank for training. The result: when an obese person starts training with weights, he lacks the muscle glycogen reserves required to train. Instead the body uses the sugar in the blood which robs the sugar flow to the brain, leaving him feeling weak and dizzy.

Q) Can't the obese person eat more carbs so he has

the fuel to train?

A) Fat people tend to store carbs as fat! In an attempt to fill their muscles up with glycogen from carbohydrates, the body stores the carbs as fat.

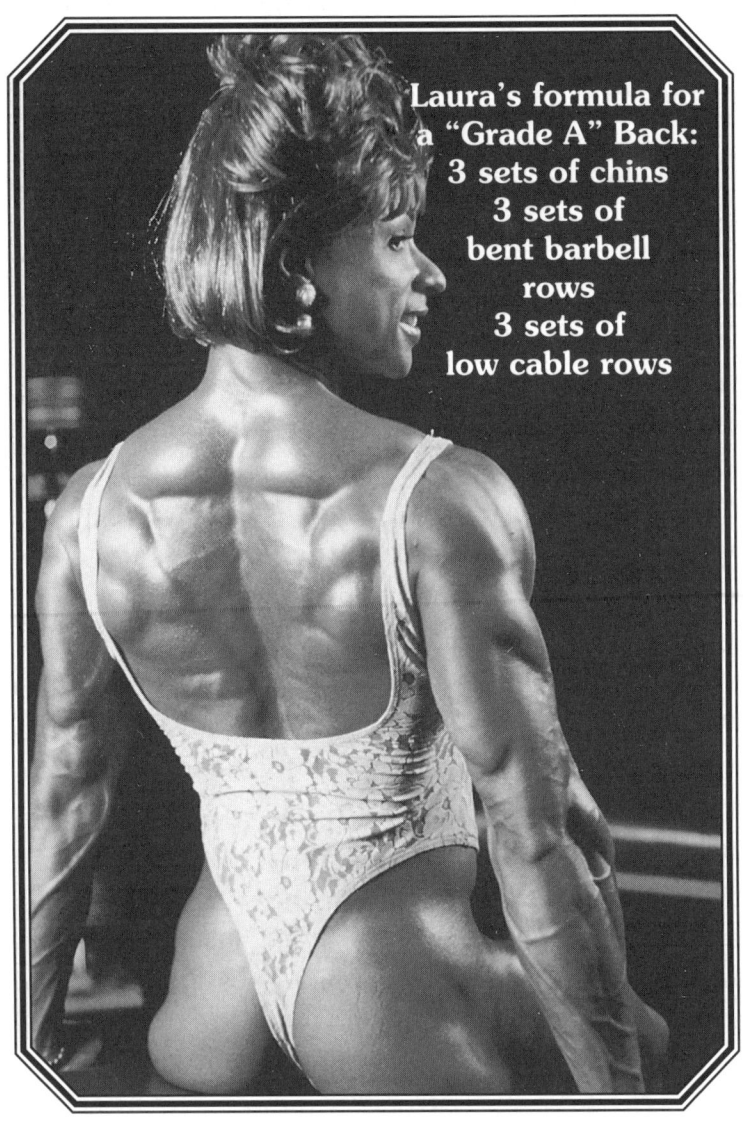

Laura's formula for a "Grade A" Back:
3 sets of chins
3 sets of bent barbell rows
3 sets of low cable rows

Q) Why can't the obese simply eat more carbs to have the fuel to train?
A) Lean people tend to store carbs as muscle glycogen. When their glycogen reserves are full, they will store all additional carbohydrates as body fat. The obese by-pass storing carbohydrates as muscle glycogen. Their carbohydrates are likely to be stored as fat instead of muscle glycogen. It's possible for an obese individual to have low muscle glycogen stores (so they have little energy to weight train) and still store carbohydrates as fat.

Q) Why do the obese store carbs as fat?
A) The higher one's body fat, the greater the release of insulin.

Q) What does high amounts of insulin do in the obese?
A) High amounts of insulin clears the carbohydrates out of the blood, and into fat stores.

Q) Please recap the exercise prescription for the obese.
A) The best exercise for the obese is aerobic exercise. The primary goal for an obese individual is fat loss.

Q) Like what?
A) Walking, stationary cycling, treadmill walking, mild stair climbing; 7 days a week at a very low to low intensity is best. One hour sessions are optimal.

Q) Why a low intensity?
A) The obese individual can not increase the intensity because as the intensity increases, his ability to complete the full hour decreases.

Q) Why an hour, why not 20 minutes.
A) It is better to lower the intensity and complete the hour than to up the intensity and complete 20 minutes. The obese do not burn a lot of fat at rest. They're **sugar burners** and lack the enzymes to burn up fat. The fuel source for aerobics is fat. By prescribing an hour session, the obese individual is **forced** to use fat as fuel. The long sessions begin to **build** the aerobic system. Specifically these sessions **increase** the enzymes to burn fat. In time, as body fat is shed through caloric expenditure, the body will have added fat burning enzymes and his body chemistry will shift from being a sugar burner at rest to a fat burner - like the lean individual.

THE FOLLOWING 11 QUESTIONS PERTAIN TO THOSE INDIVIDUALS WHO FALL INTO CATEGORY 2.

Q) What is the exercise prescription for those who fall into category 2.
A) Their time should be split between cardio work and weight training. Remember, the goal with all exercise is to alter body composition; to decrease body fat and to increase muscle mass.

Q) How much weight training and how much cardio should I do?
A) The individual in category 2 has one goal - to change his composition. However, he must perform 2 types of exercise to reach that goal. The two forms of exercise are cardiovascular training and weight training. He should **balance** the two and split his

workouts into 3 weight training sessions a week and 3 aerobic sessions a week.

Q) How **long** should his aerobic sessions be?
A) He should perform 45 to 60 minutes of aerobic activity three times a week.

Q) When should he perform the aerobics?
A) He should perform his aerobic sessions on days he does not weight train. When aerobic sessions are tagged onto the end of weight training sessions, the total length of the workouts become too long, leaving an individual susceptible to overtraining.

Q) What's the problem with overtraining?
A) When the body becomes overtrained, **overtired** really, it becomes impossible to change your body composition. Adding muscle and losing fat become nearly impossible! Overtraining releases hormones that tear down muscle tissue. When you lose muscle, your muscle to fat ratio is changed (for the worse) and less muscle translates into a slower metabolism which leads to **increases in body fat.**

Q) So I should separate my aerobic and weight training sessions and do each on different days?
A) Yes. Also, the best time to do your aerobic work is in the morning upon rising, with no food in your stomach.

Q) Why?
A) When a person eats a meal, he consumes carbohydrates. Carbohydrates breakdown in the body

as sugar and release a hormone called insulin. Insulin retards fat cells from breaking down to be used as fuel. Performing aerobics on an empty stomach will cause greater fat breakdown as there will be no insulin present to prevent or slow fat from being used.

Q) I should weight train three times a week?
A) Yes, the person falling into category 2 will carry a relatively high amount of body fat. His training goal should be to work each muscle once weekly. This can be accomplished by training on Monday, Wednesday and Friday. He can train like so:

Monday:	Chest and back
Wednesday:	Legs and calves
Friday:	Shoulders, arms and abs

On the opposite days, Tuesdays, Thursdays and Saturdays, he can perform his aerobic work in the morning on an empty stomach.

Q) But I'm more advanced. I think I should be training daily.
A) Technically, you are training daily. You are alternating aerobic work and weight training. Going into the gym to weight train daily **and** do aerobic work could lead to over training. However, an **option** is as follows. You can "exchange" your 3 one hour aerobic sessions for 6 thirty minute sessions also performed in the morning on an empty stomach. Then, **return later in the afternoon** or evening and train one bodypart. The training would look like this:

Monday:	Chest
Tuesday:	Back

Wednesday: Legs and calves
Thursday: Shoulders and abs
Friday: Arms

Rest during the weekend from weight training.

Q) If I train just one body part daily, the workouts will be extremely short.
A) That's right. Remember weight training is an anaerobic sport much like sprinting. It's characterized by explosive all out bursts in energy. It's the exact **opposite** of cardio work. The ultimate aerobic athlete is someone who "paces" himself and works for a long time at a low intensity. Bodybuilders should never pace themselves. Your workouts should be "balls to the walls" in intensity. If you train hard with all-out effort, it becomes **impossible** to train long.

If you came into the gym with me and I told you we were going to train chest and do a total of 40 sets, you would think I was crazy. Furthermore, you would "pace" yourself by using lighter weights and you would have to "hold back" and never work any set to failure.

However, if you came into the gym and I told you we were going to perform just 2 sets for chest, you would pile on as much weight as possible and take the set to failure. This type of attitude and training is a must if you want to add muscle. Use heavy weights, take the sets to failure, never pace yourself and do not do a lot of sets - you can't if you are truly pushing yourself.

Q) So I should choose brief workouts over longer ones.
A) Exactly, if long workouts were the key to adding mass, the workouts that would be best would be the

ones that included the "most amount of sets." Surely training is more complicated than simple volume work.

THE FOLLOWING 16 QUESTIONS PERTAIN TO THOSE INDIVIDUALS WHO FALL INTO CATEGORY 3.

Q) What type of training should I do if I fall in category 3?
A) The person of category 3 status also wants to alter his body composition - increase muscle and lose body fat. Since he has much less fat than the person in category 1 or 2, he should focus on adding muscle mass **first.** His **secondary** focus should be to shed and lose fat. Therefore he should do more weight training than aerobic training.

Q) How much aerobic work?
A) Three to four 20 to 30 minutes sessions a week is plenty. Anymore will make muscle building more difficult.

Q) That sounds contradictory. Why is the person who falls in category 2 doing so much more aerobic work. Won't it interfere with muscle growth?
A) Possibly, but is is important for him to lose fat (since he carries a lot of it) and to add muscle. You could say his goal is **twofold;** shed fat and add muscle. Your goal is different. Since you have less fat to lose, your goal is to build muscle first and foremost and then or secondary, to focus on fat loss.

Q) How should I weight train in category 3?

A) Focus on "building and resting." That means you should stress training harder with heavier weights. Remember, the harder you train (heavier weights taking your sets to failure), you must perform fewer total sets and make sure you recover between workouts. Because you will be doing less aerobic activity, you will have more energy to channel towards your weight training. A good split may be the two on one off training schedule where you rest after each two successive training days.

Q) If I'm to do 3 or 4 twenty to thirty minute aerobic sessions each week, when and where is the best time to schedule them?

A) You have two choices to schedule your aerobics with your weight training here are the two ways:

Day 1: AM: cardio 20-30 minutes   PM: train back & abs
Day 2: AM: cardio 20-30 minutes   PM:train chest & shoulders
Day 3: REST
Day 4: no cardio   PM: train legs & calves
Day 5: AM cardio (optional)*   PM: train arms
Day 6: AM cardio   PM: rest
Day 7: REPEAT ENTIRE CYCLE

* The exercise prescription calls for 3 to 4 aerobic sessions weekly. Above, you should start with 3 sessions, if body fat is still a problem (ie. it is not coming off, increase the cardio sessions to 4 per week) If you are not losing fat and are performing aerobic work 4 times a week, you must concentrate on your diet and food intake. It's possible you are not following the right type of diet. Any fat burning effects from your cardio work is being sabotaged by your food intake.

Q) The obese should be doing long and low intensity aerobics. What intensity should I follow while I am on the treadmill?

A) For those who fall in category 3, you should increase the intensity to 70% of your maximum heart rate and maintain it for the full 20 to 30 minutes.

Q) Why an increase in intensity.

A) Recall the obese are **not** good fat burners. They burn sugar and when they train with weights, they quickly become dizzy and weak as sugar is rapidly used up leaving the brain starving for fuel. They perform long slow aerobic sessions at a lower intensity to **force** their body to build enzymes to burn fat. If their intensity is too high, they would never be able to complete the full hour. The goal is simple: "kick start" the fat burning process.

Someone who is not obese, (the person in category 2) yet carries extra body fat can train with weights to add muscle and do cardio to burn fat. He has the ability to burn fat and he doesn't feel faint while weight training. He can do both forms of exercise and get results simultaneously - he can add muscle with weight training and shed fat through aerobic work. The net change is a drastic alteration in body composition - the amount of muscles mass increases while the amount of fat he carries decreases.

Generally, the person with even less fat (category 3) is in better "shape" to begin with, so he can push himself harder by increasing **both** aerobic intensity and weight training intensity. How does he increase aerobic intensity? By working at a 70% heart rate. How does he increase weight training intensity? By increasing the load on the muscle via heavier weights.

Q) I'm a male with 13% body fat. By your assessment, I fall into category 3. How much weight training and aerobics should I do?
A) Those in category 3 should again, like those in category 2, focus on adding lean body mass first. Aerobics and diet must be emphasized to lose, inhibit and control body fat.

Q) What is the goal of each set?
A) The goal in each set you perform is to cause the muscle to fail in the 6 to 12 rep range. If you can just barely complete rep #6 through #12 on your own, you have accomplished your immediate goal and caused muscle failure.

If you can perform **more than** 12 reps, the weight is too light, and if you **fail to reach** 6 reps, the weight is to heavy for you.

Q) How long should I wait before I do my next set?
A) Recall the goal; to cause muscle failure on each set. Therefore, you should **not** try to "speed" through your workout. Rest intervals of one minute are a minimum for smaller bodyparts like biceps, triceps, abs, and calves. However, larger muscles like chest, and shoulders may require longer rest between sets and the largest muscles like back and legs could require 3 minutes in between sets. As a rule of thumb; rest long enough to accomplish 2 things. First, allow your heart rate to return to close to resting levels. Second, rest long enough so that you regain the strength and confidence to perform another heavy set - like the one you just finished.

Q) What's my heart rate got to do with weight training?
A) Many who work to quickly through their workouts, fatigue early because their entire body is tired. The body as a **unit** can become tired and fatigued during a set if your heart rate did not have a chance to return to normal. Therefore you stop doing a set because you are tired, fatigued, out of breath, or your lungs could be "burning" (this often occurs while training legs). The only reason to stop doing a set is due to **local** muscle failure - you couldn't complete another rep.

Q) I thought cutting down on rest between sets is a way to increase the intensity of my workout.
A) Actually, it causes **decreases** in intensity.

Q) Explain that to me.
A) Intensity in bodybuilding is primarily measured by how effectively you taxed your muscles in one workout. The **weight** (or load) is directly correlated with how much **tension** is placed on the muscles. The more tension, the greater the "intensity!" Intensity has **nothing** to do with cutting down on rest intervals.

I'll give you an example. Which of the two below is more "intense"
1) 3 sets of 10 reps with 100 pounds
2) 1 set of 10 reps 100 pounds, followed by 1 set of 10 reps with 85 pounds, followed by 1 set with 80 pounds. The answer is 1. By resting longer, 1 can perform each set with maximal weight while 2, who "speeds" through his workout with short rest intervals,

fails to place the maximum amount of tension on the muscle at each set.

Here is another way to explain rest intervals. If you performed a heavy set of 10 reps on the bench press, I would expect you to be able to perform a second set of 10 reps with the same heavy weight if you rested sufficiently and long enough before attempting your second set.

However, if you performed that heavy set of 10 reps, waited just 30 to 45 seconds in between sets, before trying the same weight again for your second set, you would not be able to complete 10 reps.

Q) Can I expect more progress by continually changing the angles of the exercises (on each bodypart)?
A) No. Many beginners make the mistake of training too fast and not resting sufficiently between sets. Another mistake is believing that changing angles contributes to greater physique changes. To dispel the "angle myth" you must understand how muscles contract and grow. When a muscle is worked, **nearly** the entire muscle comes into play. For example, on bench presses, the entire chest is worked; the "upper" "mid" and "lower" pecs come into play. As you approach muscle fatigue in the 6 to 12 rep range, all the individual fibers come into play in all parts of the muscle. At the point where you struggle and can no longer complete another rep, all the muscle fibers in the chest are activated. The result is you obtain **complete** chest development from this one exercise! Those who prescribe changing angles don't really grasp the above. They believe changing angles will

cause more muscle contraction and more muscle development.

Q) Then what does changing the angles do?
A) Varying angles changes the direction of the stress upon the muscle. So, changing from flat benches to inclines places more stress on the upper pecs. However, you will not get maximal chest development even in the upper pec region unless you take the set to failure.

Many mistakenly believe varying angles will recruit all the muscle fibers of a muscle. The physiological truth is that all muscle fibers of a working muscle will come into play if the tension (weight) is great enough to cause total muscle fiber recruitment. It is possible to train a muscle from every conceivable angle and not obtain total development if the tension is not great.

Q) It's possible to fail to grow even if I change the angles and exercises?
A) Yes. Changing angles will only be effective if you take exercises to failure.

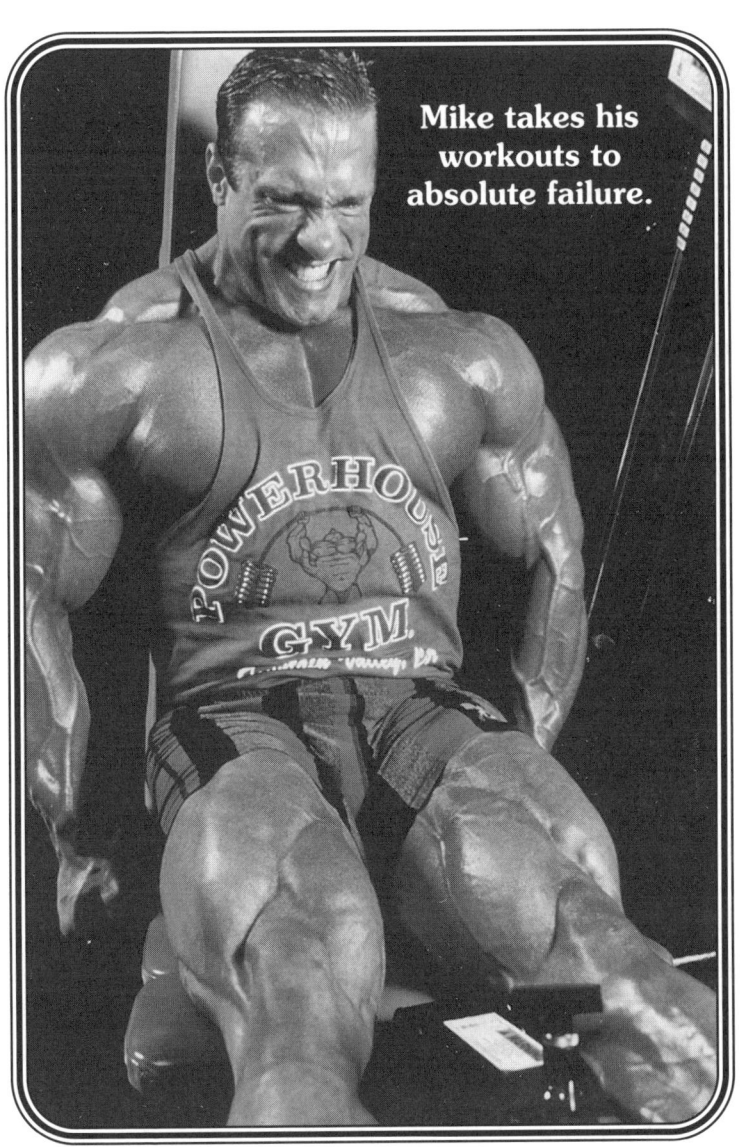

Q) If I a person is around 8 to 12% body fat, what should be the training goal?
A) Most bodybuilders or those who look like bodybuilders should aspire to maintain lower levels of body fat. I think 8 to 12% is a very acceptable number. If you are a male and carry a relatively low level of body fat, you will have to put more into your training and diet to get good results.

Since you are already pretty lean, there is no reason to waste your time and energy on aerobics. You should focus on adding mass and preventing fat accumulation **by paying strict attention to your diet.**

Q) How should I train?
A) The longer you have been bodybuilding, the harder you can "push" yourself in the gym. The catch-22 is this: your ability to recover from your training is not significantly greater than the first year you began training. As a rule of thumb, the longer you have been training and the harder you train, the more rest you need between workouts to fully recover! You must be careful of overtraining.

Therefore, you should stick to a program that allows you to train **as often as possible while obtaining as much rest as possible.** Here is where individuality comes into the equation as some will be able to recover faster than others. Remember, if you rarely see increases in strength or you are not growing, chances are good you need more rest. Here are 3 training schedules. It is impossible for me to recommend one to each and every reader. You must choose which one works best for you. All three call for working each muscle just once each week.

3 days on 1 day off	
Day 1	train: chest and triceps
Day 2	train: legs and calves
Day 3	train: back and abs
Day 4	rest
Day 5	train: shoulders and biceps
Day 6	Rest, repeat
4 days on 2 days off	
Day 1	train: chest and biceps or chest and shoulders
Day 2	train: back and abs or legs and calves
Day 3	train: legs and calves or arms
Day 4	train: shoulders and triceps or back and abs
Day 5 & 6	Rest, repeat
2 days on 1 day off	
Day 1	chest and biceps
Day 2	back and abs
Day 3	Rest
Day 4	legs and calves
Day 5	shoulders and triceps Rest, then repeat

Q) Should I always stay within the 6 to 12 rep range?

A) No. Although muscles seem to grow best in the 6 to 12 rep range, we know heavy weights performed in the 1 to 5 rep range will increase muscle strength with less emphasis on building size. You should alter you training after every 8 weeks and perform only sets of 3 to 5 reps. Performing lower reps with higher weights will increase your strength.

Q) But I thought the 1 to 5 rep range causes mostly increases in strength with very little increases in muscle mass.

A) True. You will be performing 2 weeks of low reps with more weight to build up your strength. Then you will return to your normal rep range of 6 to 12 reps. Working in the lower range will increase your strength and you will be able to "borrow" this strength improvement when you go back to your 6 to 12 rep sets. In essence, you are taking a 2 week break from 6 to 12 reps to work in the lower rep ranges to improve your strength. Then you will return to the 6 to 12 rep range and you will be able to **lift more weight.** The greater tension you can put on your muscles in the 6 to 12 rep range, the greater your ability to work all the muscle fibers in each muscle and cause maximum muscle growth.

Q) Why no aerobics?
A) Aerobics does not build muscle. If you are already lean or on the lean side forget about them! While they do burn body fat, they have a negative aspect - they zap your ability to recover from your weight training workouts. Your body only has a certain amount of recovery ability. If you are training alone, and not doing aerobic work, your body will grow. When you add aerobics, which **requires** energy, you rob your body of its full potential to recover!

Q) How do I control body fat without cardio work?
A) You can control fat by training **hard!** You do not have to do aerobic exercise to be lean.

Q) But aerobics burns fat and weight training does not burn fat?

A) You are right, weight training burns sugar as fuel and the sugar is derived from carbohydrates foods. These carbs are stored within muscles as muscle glycogen.

Even though weight training does not burn fat, it is the best fat burner, better than aerobics, in the long run. (for relatively lean people).

Q) Explain this! How can an activity that does not burn fat be the best fat burning exercise?
A) The answer lies in **metabolism!** First, an individual who is relatively lean burns fat at rest. Specifically, 2/3 of all the calories you burn up while sitting comes from fat. Some of this fat is derived from dietary fat that you may have eaten and the rest from stored body fat. 1/3 of the calories you burn at rest comes from sugars. The sugar comes from sugar that is floating around in the blood from eating carbohydrates and from muscle glycogen stores. At rest, a lean person burns more fat than sugar!

Q) How many calories do I burn at rest?
A) The amount of calories you burn at rest is called your basal metabolic rate or BMR. BMR is the amount of calories you need each day at rest - doing absolutely nothing at all. Technically, it is the amount of calories your body needs to sustain life; to pump blood, and maintain the heart beat, nervous system, etc.

Q) How do I know what my BMR is?
A) Simply find your lean body mass via a percent body fat measurement test. (total weight - fat weight = lean

body mass). Then "tag" a zero at the end. For example if your lean body mass is 188 pounds, your BMR is 1880 calories (188 + zero = 1880).

Therefore, a person with a lean body mass of 188 pounds needs 1880 calories a day at rest.

Q) I still don't quite understand how weight training burns fat.
A) The more muscle you have, the more calories you need each day at rest. Adding muscle can increase the BMR! And since fat is the fuel for a resting lean body, weight training and the muscle built as a result, increases calorie needs and fat burning.

Interestingly, it is tremendously difficult to **exceed**

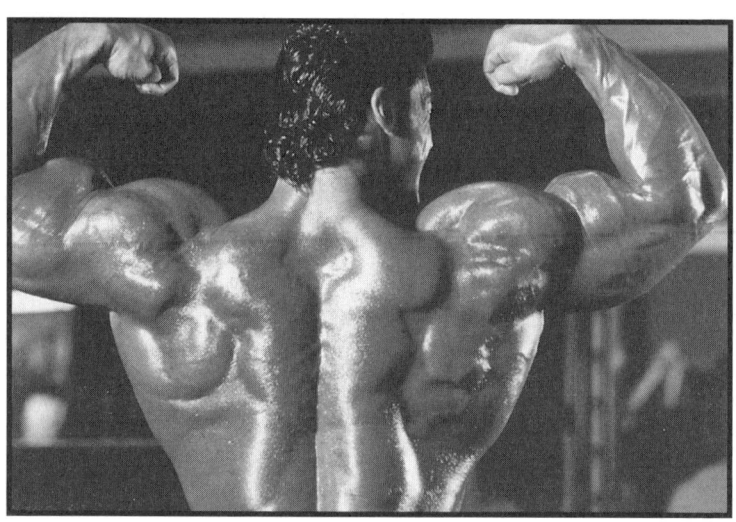

Low body fat levels are achieved with a high metabolism.

your BMR via exercise. For example, each minute of aerobic exercise (which uses fat as fuel) burns about 7 to 10 calories. Two full non stop hours of stair climbing may burn off 1200 calories, a far cry from your BMR. While aerobic work burns fat as fuel, your caloric needs from your BMR always exceed the total calories you can burn through exercise! Plus, resting muscles use fat as fuel!

Q) But weight training doesn't stimulate my metabolism like aerobics can.
A) Wrong again. In fact weight training has the greatest effect on your metabolism. Let me explain. Many who do aerobics are under the impression that they burn more calories for hours and hours **after** the aerobic workout. In reality the metabolic "kick" associated with aerobic exercise is very small.

When you do aerobic work, you burn calories, most of these calories are derived from fat - either dietary fat or body fat stores. Upon completing the aerobic work, your body will burn more calories at rest for an hour or two following the training. Here is an example.

A person with a BMR of 1880 calories a day will burn about 78 calories an hour (1880 divided by 24 hours). When he does an hour worth of aerobics, he burns a total of 600 calories (10 calories a minute x 60 minutes.) If he returns to a resting state, literally not moving for the rest of the day, we can safely assume he will burn 2480 calories for the day:

1880 BMR
+600 burned through exercise
2480 total calories burned for the day.

The aerobic advocate will argue the BMR is elevated after the aerobic work, so he burns "a lot more calories even at rest - all day long". That statement is simply false. The person will burn 10 to

15% more calories for an hour or two **only** after training aerobically. Instead of burning 78 calories an hour at rest, he will burn 10 to 15% more for just 1 to 2 hours or 86 to 91 calories at rest in the two post exercise hours. After two hours, he will go back to burning 78 calories each hour.

Q) How is weight training different?
A) Weight training causes micro tears in the muscle. Micro tears are a form of trauma. **All** trauma increases the metabolic rate. In fact, severe trauma can **double** your BMR!

A person who trains correctly, in the 6 to 12 rep range, and takes his sets to failure will inflict micro tears upon the muscle. These tears will increase the BMR from 10 to 20% for up to 24 hours. Here is an example to illustrate the point.

BMR= 1880 calories a day.

A bodybuilder trains for one hour and burns roughly half the amount of calories an aerobic athlete uses in the same hour. (Super hard trainers can burn up to 500 calories an hour.) If the bodybuilder does not move a single muscle for the rest of the day - he goes home to bed, we can expect him to burn 2180 calories for the day.

Here's the catch: he wakes up the next day and has burned far greater than 2180 calories. **Muscle tears increase the BMR by up to 30% for up to 24 hours.** The BMR has shifted from 1880 to 2444 calories.

1880 calories is the BMR x .30% increase due to muscle trauma.

The new BMR is 2444 calories.

    1880
    x.30
    2440 calories are used in the coming 24 hours at rest.

Now, add the 300 calories that are burned during the weight training session and the grand total is 2740 calories.

Overall, here's the difference:

<u>Weight</u> <u>Trainer</u>   VS.   <u>Aerobic</u> <u>Trainer</u>
2740 calories   2440 calories

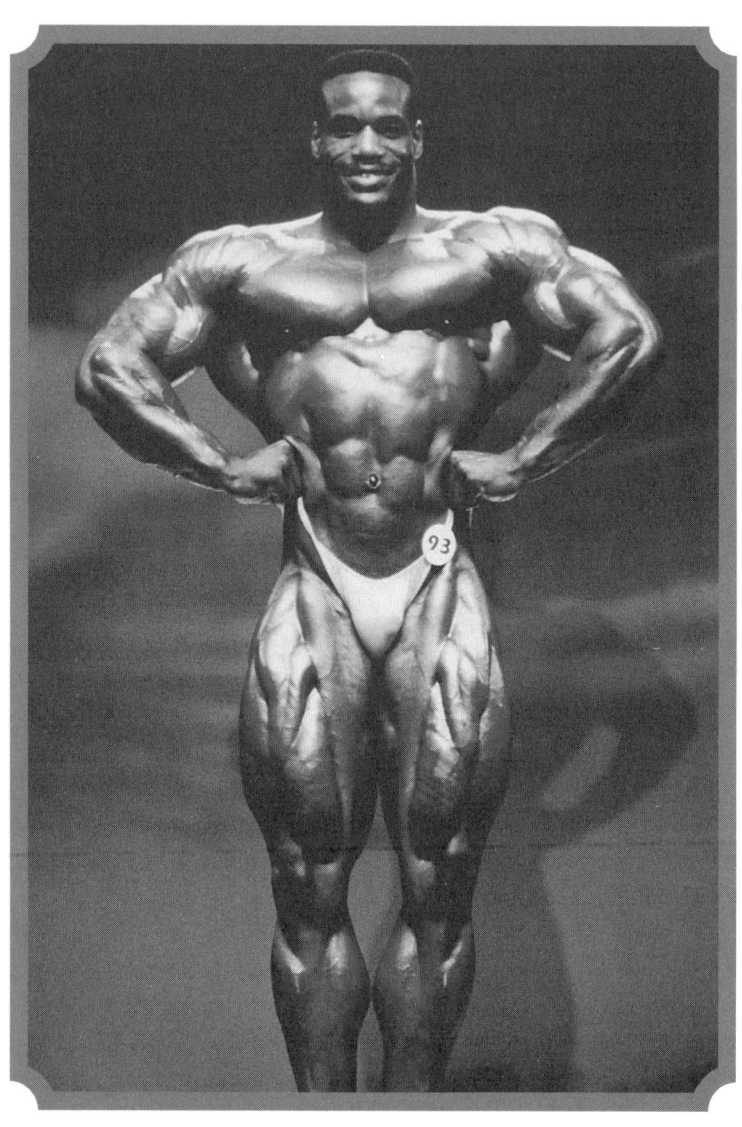

Chris Cormier relies on a reduced calorie diet & moderate cardio sessions to rip up.

Q) How do I know if I need cardio exercise?
A) Refer to your category on page 47. Another easy way is to generalize. If you are lean or if you have a fast metabolism, you do not need to do any aerobic work!

If you are moderately lean or have a moderate to good metabolism, then you should do aerobics. Three times a week in the morning on an empty stomach would be helpful in controlling body fat levels. Each session should be roughly 20 to 30 minutes.

If you have a slow metabolism or a high amount of body fat, you should do 4 aerobic sessions weekly in the morning on an empty stomach. Each session should last up to 45 minutes.

If you are obese, you should perform low intensity aerobics and no weight training. The goal for the very heavy individual is to force the body to lose fat and to increase the total number of fat burning enzymes in the body. This can be accomplished through low intensity aerobic sessions on a daily basis. First thing in the morning is still a wise idea, but anytime is fine - as long as you do it!

Q) What is the setpoint theory in weight loss?
A) Set point is your individual point where diet and exercise will no longer make you leaner. For many the set point may be higher than for others. Two heavy set individuals could embark on a diet and exercise program and one may lower his level of body fat much lower than the other. The difference in their end result is due to their setpoint.

Q) What causes set point?
A) Set point, in general, is associated with genetics.

Q) How can I over come a set point?
A) To understand setpoint, you must understand the very nature of aerobic exercise. Aerobics burns fat as fuel. If you are obese and perform an hour of cardio work today, you can expect to lose or burn off approximately 600 calories of energy. Since 3500 calories expended is approximately equal to one pound of fat, you could expect to lose/expend 3600 calories or 1 pound of body fat in 6 days. (6 x 600 = 3600).

If you perform this same aerobic work, 6 times a week for one year, you will **not** lose 52 pounds of body fat! The reason is this: the body adapts to calorie expenditure via aerobic work by **accommodation.** We know low calorie diets do not work in the long run because the body accommodates to the calorie reduction by slowing its metabolism. The truth is, the body works the same during caloric expenditure. The more aerobic work you do, in the long run, the fewer calories you expend! This makes aerobic work as the sole source of body fat control futile in the long run. The more you do the less you burn. You reach your set point as it becomes harder and harder to shed body fat.

Q) Can't I lose more fat by simply decreasing my caloric intake.
A) Not really. Cutting calories backfires. The more you cut, the more your body fights to hold onto its fat stores as reducing calories signals the "starvation response" where the body tries to "survive" and hold onto its calorie reservoir - known as fat stores. A high amount of aerobics to expend calories coupled with a strict diet to omit calories leads to a metabolic slowdown and you'll only be able to get as lean as your genetics, (your set point), dictates.

Q) How can I overcome my set point?
A) The only way to overcome your set point is to add muscle mass through progressive weight training. Weight training is the exact **opposite** to aerobic training. The longer you weight train, the more muscle you build. The more muscle you have, the more calories you burn in each workout! It takes more fuel to move around a 185 pound body than a 175 pound body. Furthermore, the more muscle you can add to your body, the greater your metabolism! Only muscle mass increases your metabolism. Aerobics, since it does not add muscle to the body, does not really increase your metabolism.

Q) What do you mean by metabolism.
A) By metabolism, I mean basal metabolism. Your basal metabolism is the amount of calories you require in a 24 hour period if you do absolutely nothing at all but lie in bed or sit in front of the television.

Q) How is metabolism related to weight training, but not aerobic exercise?
A) Weight training build muscle and aerobic training does not. Muscles require fuel at rest. The more muscle a person has, the more fuel he needs at rest.

Q) Can you give me an example?
A) Sure. You can guestimate your basal metabolism, the amount of calories your body needs at complete rest in a day, by finding your lean body mass.

Q) How do I find lean body mass?
A) Get a body composition by calipers or electro impedence. Either test will tell you two things. What part of you (in pounds) is fat and how much of you (in

pounds) is muscle and bones. If you are 200 pounds and are 10% body fat, you have 180 pounds of muscle and 20 pounds of body fat.

To find basal metabolism "tag" a zero to the end of your lean body weight - the part of you that is muscle and bones. A person with a lean body weight of 180 "tags" a zero to become 1800. Therefore, he needs 1800 calories a day at complete rest.

As you can see, a person with 12 pounds of lean body mass needs 1200 calories a day at complete rest and a person with a lean body weight of 155 needs 1550 calories a day at complete rest.

Q) So weight training can "re-set" my metabolism.
A) Exactly. But there's more. When a person with a ton of muscle peddles a bike for 30 minutes, he burns a lot more total calories than the person with a lot less muscle. It takes **more fuel** in the form of calories to move a big body around than a smaller one.

Imagine a 250 pound man and his wife weighing 120 pounds doing aerobics each day for 45 minutes. Both perform the exercise at 70% of the maximum heart rate and both use the treadmill and walk side by side. In each session, the male will burn **radically more calories and fat** than the female due to his large size. It simply takes him more fuel to do the same work. Now picture a motorcycle and a huge Lincoln Navigator both driving along the highway, side by side, for 8 hours at 55 miles per hour. Although they both arrive at their final destination at the same time, the smaller motorcycle may require 5 gallons of fuel to replace the fuel he burned during the trip while the larger Lincoln that weighs dramatically more may require 18 gallons of fuel. The take home message:

adding muscle mass allows you to burn more fat ***when you do your aerobics.***

Q) Explain the progressive overload principle.
A) The overload principle states that muscle growth can continue as long as the muscles are continually or "progressively" overloaded. A beginner, someone who enters the gym for the very first time, can overload his muscles with the lightest of weights. In order to continue to make progress, he must systematically ("progressively") increase the load (the stress) on the muscle.

Q) What is the stress?
A) The stress for the beginner is the weight he uses or it is the total number of sets he uses. Both lead to overload. The same two factors are true for an intermediate and advanced athlete.

Q) Then what should I use to progressively overload my muscles. Should I add more weight or should I add more sets?
A) **Beginners** should strive to increase the number of sets you do first.

Q) Why?
A) Adding more sets is the **easiest** way to progressively overload the muscles.

Q) How do I know when to stop increasing my sets?
A) You should do no more than 2 to 3 good sets per exercise for a total of 6 for biceps and triceps, 9 for shoulders, 9 for back 6 to 8 for chest, 9 for legs including your hamstrings and 6 for calves. This recommendation if for beginners to intermediates.

Q) Can advanced athletes do more sets.

A) Yes, but there is a point of diminishing returns. Advanced athletes can do up to 9 for biceps or triceps, 12 to 16 for legs, 12 for chest, 12 for shoulders, 12 to 14 for back and 9 for calves. Beware: More may not be better.

Q) Why not more sets?
A) If you try to do too many sets, the poundages you use fall.

Q) When should I up my weight as a way to progressively overload the muscles?
A) Although you should always strive to bump up the weight you use to overload the muscles, it is easier to increase the sets first, then once you are performing the recommended amount of sets as a beginner or intermediate), you should strive to add more and more weight as a means to progressively overload the muscles.

Q) What is relative overload?
A) Relative overload is when a bodybuilder does too many sets in hopes of achieving progressive overload. Workouts that are too long in volume, that include too many sets for each bodypart, definitely stress the muscles. The problem is excessive sets, doing too much, will prevent you from using the maximum poundages you could potentially use on each set. It is very possible to "feel" like your working hard, when in fact, you are simply tiring your self out with too much training **without** using maximum weights. You can not fulfill your genetic potential unless you are able to reach your strength potential in the 6 to 12 rep range. Never forget: strength is correlated with muscle size!

    The second problem with relative overload and doing too many sets is you end up tired and simply overtrained. Recall, overtraining kills muscle recovery and muscle growth! It's more difficult to overtrain doing fewer sets but putting more effort into each set than from doing volume work. Plus, doing fewer sets allows you to train heavier.

Q) How long should I take to prepare for a bodybuilding contest?
A) The longer the better! These days, even novice competitions are tremendously competitive. The condition athletes achieve is astounding. Allow yourself 20 weeks to prepare if you are carrying a lot of fat, 16 weeks if you are muscular but soft in certain areas, and 8 to 13 weeks if you are in good shape and have a good metabolism.

Q) What tips can you give me for my first show?
A) Start early! This takes a lot of the guess work out of contest preparation. If you make mistakes, it's always nice to have extra time to make corrections, to get back on track without panicking.

Many panicked bodybuilders make every conceivable diet, training and cardio mistake in the book and end up looking just plain bad the day of the show. Second, do not overdiet! Many novices overdiet as they do not realize that a competition ready physique is the result of **retaining muscle while shedding excess fat.** Instead, they believe its possible to look like a bodybuilder by putting themselves on an overly strict diet which catabolizes muscle tissue and leaves the bodybuilder looking flat or soft. The third suggestion is to perform only moderate amounts of cardio work. Most bodybuilders seem to go overboard on cardio before contests which leave them overtrained and flat. Any bodybuilder who has ever competed with "flat" muscles the day of the show knows he would have been better off had he come into the show not fully dieted down, but full. A contest winning physique can never be flat, it must be full. Avoid becoming flat with a good contest plan. Try 16 to 20 weeks of preparations, don't over diet, and include moderate amounts of cardio work - 4 45 minutes sessions each week would be the maximum amount most will need. Finally, look for small changes in your physique from week to week. Nobody can get into shape overnight. Be patient.

Q) I fall into the 20 week-prep category. Should I use more high rep sets?
A) No. Depending on what kind of shape you are in and take a full 20 weeks to prepare or ten weeks, you should avoid high reps.

Q) Why?
A) High reps do not burn more fat. In fact **all** weight training uses sugar derived from the carbohydrate food you eat, as fuel.

Q) How many reps should I use pre-contest?
A) It's best to perform the **rep range** that gave you the muscle you have in the first place! In fact, try to lift the same weights pre-contest as you did in the "off season".

If you decrease your weights, you are decreasing the stimulus that caused the muscles to grow. It's as simple as this: remove the **stimulus** and you will remove your ability to grow or **preserve** and hold your muscles while in the pre-contest phase.

Never use your weight training as a tool to burn fat. Weight training serves a specific purpose; to build muscle and to hold muscle. Use your **diet** and **cardio** exercise to accomplish its intended purpose; to burn off unwanted body fat!

Q) I thought a higher rep range can help shape a muscle.
A) This is a myth. Your shape depends almost exclusively on your genetics. If you have a short bicep or tricep, you can not change this (the muscle's origin point and attachment) through special rep ranges or angles. Concentrate on building as much mass as possible and your "shape" will fall where it may. Don't think for a minute that Flex Wheeler could spoil his incredible shape by training in the wrong rep range or by doing different angles. He has a naturally small waist, small joints, and round shaped muscles. Likewise, someone with a Dorian Yates looking body can never alter it to look like Flex Wheeler's.

Q) What type of training split should I follow pre-contest?
A) This depends on your own personal ability to recover fully from your workouts. Some can train more frequently than others.
    I like the 2 day on 1 day rest split. It may prevent you from overtraining, a common pre-contest mistake. The split looks like so:

Day 1:	train	chest and shoulders (abs, optional)
Day 2:	train	legs and calves
Day 3:	rest	completely
Day 4:	train	back and abs
Day 5:	train	arms (calves, optional)

Q) What about the cardio?
A) Cardio can be performed on days 1, 2, 4, or 5. in the morning, on an empty stomach to maximize fat burning. Then, you should return to the gym later in the day or in the evening to do your training.

Q) How much cardio should I do?
A) For competition, you should always start with 3 to 4 times a week and only 20 minutes at a time.

Q) Why such a small amount?
A) For 2 reasons. 1) Too much too soon may zap your recovery ability so it becomes hard to train with the same big, heavy weights that built your body in the first place. 2) Why do 4 times a week for an hour when a mild aerobic program will do the job.

Start with the smallest amount to cause fat loss. Check your progress through skin calipers and photos. If you are seeing steady results (small changes) continue with the same aerobic schedule. If you stop seeing progress, you can systematically up your cardio work.

Q) How much is the maximum amount of cardio I should do before competing?
A) Build your pre-contest aerobic work slowly from 3 or 4 times for 20 minutes to 3 to 4 times for 30 minutes, then 3 to 4 times for 40 minutes. If you have to do more than 4 times a week at 45 minutes per clip, you will be making yourself very susceptible to overtraining and you will lack the energy to train hard with weights. As a result of too much cardio work, your muscles can loose their fullness, their "rugged" look.

Higher intensity aerobics burns more total calories than lower intensity aerobics. The bodybuilder hoping to get as lean as possible should stick with higher intensity cardio. While its true, really high intensity cardio, closer to 80% of your heart rate will cause a shift where the body may burn some muscle glycogen, the net effect of high intensity cardio is the great calorie burn and more fat loss. The confusion lies in the percentages. I call them "margins". A low intensity 40 minute session may burn as few as 250 calories with 90% coming from fat, the remaining from glycogen (stored sugar). A very high intensity session may burn 400 to 500 calories with 80% from fat and 20% coming from glycogen. The benefit of high intensity, aside from more calories burned, you really do burn more fat calories as 80% of 500 is 400 calories of fat where as 90% of 250 is only 225 calories of fat.

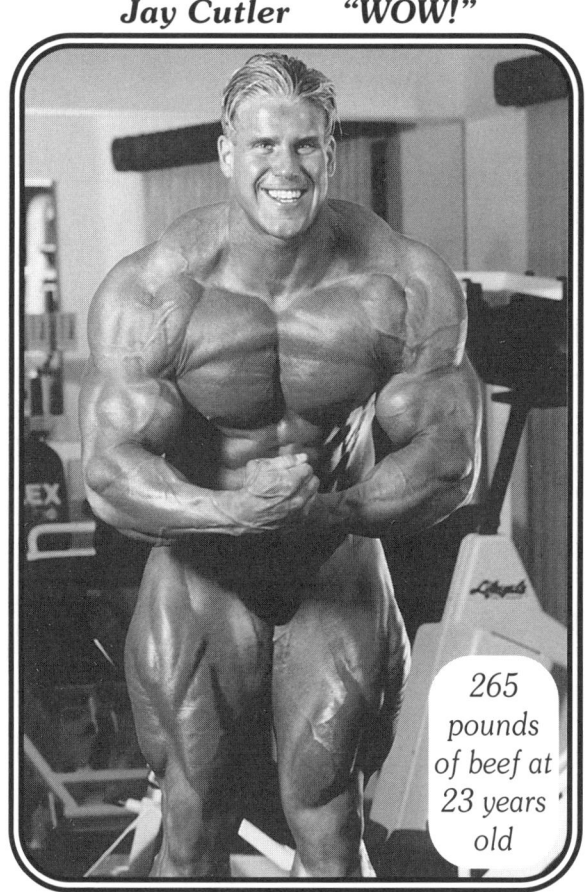

Jay Cutler   **"WOW!"**

265 pounds of beef at 23 years old

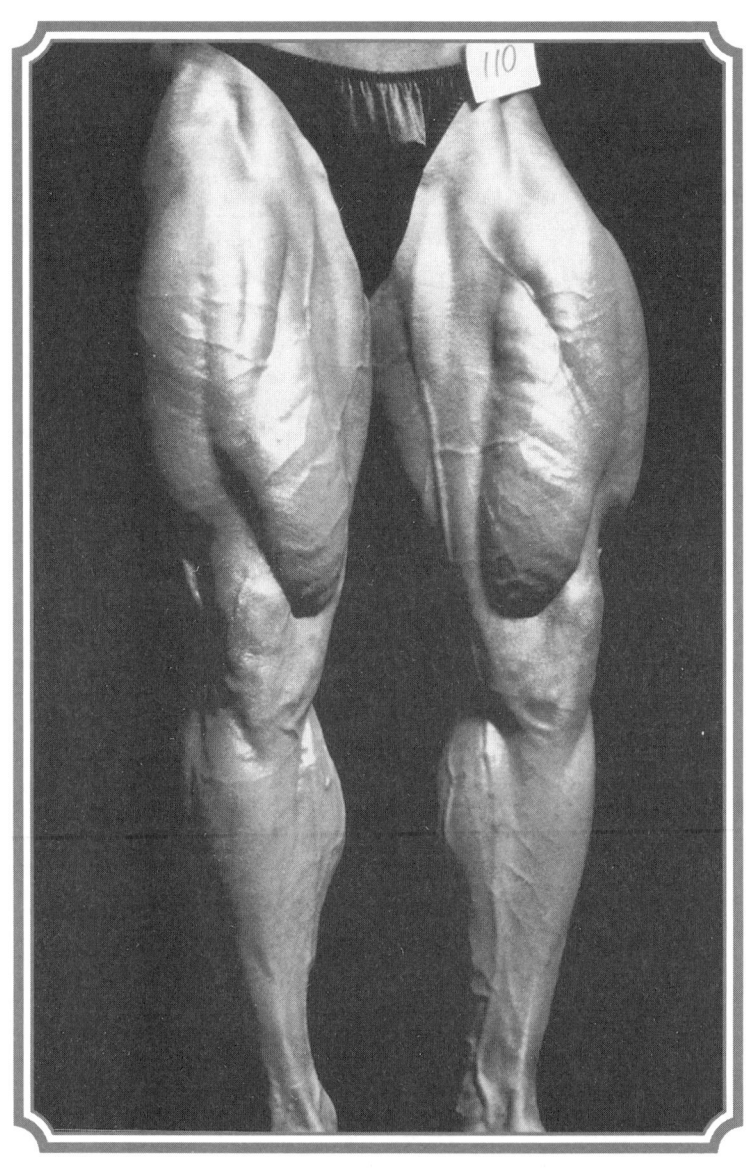

Paul "Quadzilla" DeMayo's legs weren't built with light weights and high-reps.

Nutrition Questions

Q) What is a calorie?
A) A calorie is a measuring unit, much like an inch or a meter is a way of measuring.

Q) What does a calorie measure?
A) A calorie measures how much energy is produced in the body from foods we eat.

Q) What do calories do?
A) They provide us with fuel to, in the case of a bodybuilder or aerobic athlete, work - to exercise.

Q) What is body fat?
A) Body fat is a storage location. When you consume more fuel in the form of calories than you require (to do work) the extra fuel is stored as body fat.

Q) How many calories does a person require each day.
A) That depends on two things. First, it is dependent on the amount of muscle you carry. Second, calorie

requirements are dependent on your level of activity. People with a lot of muscle require a lot of calories and people who do a lot of physical activity also need a **lot** of calories. A big muscular person who is very active will need even more fuel.

Q) How can I figure out the amount of calories I need daily?
A) That's a bit tough. However, we can easily find the amount of calories you need **at rest** each day. The amount of fuel you need at rest is closely related to the amount of muscle you carry. The amount of calories you need at rest in a 24 hour period is called your **basal metabolism** (BM)

BM can be found in two quick steps.
1) Find your lean body mass (LBM) via a skin caliper
2) Add a zero to the end of the LBM

Q) Give me an example.
A) Ok, your weight is 200 pounds and your body fat is 10%. We determine 10% of you is fat and 90% of you is muscle. Your muscle weight is your LBM. 90% of 200 pounds is 180 so your BM is 1800 calories a day.

Q) What's the 1800 mean?
A) You need 1800 calories daily to maintain your body weight if you do not move. If you ate 1800 calories and walked around all day, you could expect to lose lean body weight. You'd lose muscle as 1800 calories is only enough fuel to maintain your muscle weight **at complete rest.**

Q) What are carbohydrate foods?
A) "Carbo" foods like potatoes, whole grain breads, rice, pasta yams, oatmeal, fruits and vegetables all break down into sugar in the body. This sugar is referred to as "blood sugar" or "blood glucose"

Q) Is there a difference between these carbohydrate foods?
A) Yes, the **speed** at which they breakdown into the blood as "blood sugar" varies from carbohydrate to carbohydrate food.

Q) Can the body store carbohydrates?
A) Yes, carbohydrates can be stored in the muscle to be used later if the body lacks sugar. The storage "tank" for carbohydrates is known as muscle and liver glycogen.

Q) If I miss a meal what happens?
A) When sugar levels in the blood fall, muscle glycogen levels fall in the muscles. The muscles will give up some glycogen into the blood to keep your "blood sugar level" normal.

Q) I heard the more carbohydrates you eat, the better your workout.
A) Your on the right track. The fuel source for weight training is sugar. This sugar comes from the carbo foods you ate. If you have sugar in the blood from a recent carbo intake, your muscles can use that as fuel. When the sugar in the blood begins to fall, the body "shifts gears", and taps into muscle glycogen.

Q) Why doesn't the body continue to use blood sugar as fuel?
A) If your muscles use up too much sugar from the blood, you'd feel weak, and possibly faint. Something else besides your working muscles use sugar as fuel... the brain! Your brain relies on sugar as fuel. So, the body protects itself by "shifting" gears and tapping glycogen as fuel.

Q) So it's a good idea to pound the carbs as they are my fuel source for weight training.
A) There's a problem. Your body has limited glycogen stores. The more muscle you have, the greater your ability to store muscle glycogen. However, once glycogen stores are full, **all excess carbs will be stored as fat.** Carbohydrates, when eaten above what you need will cause fat storage.

Q) What about insulin. I hear a lot about it but I'm confused.
A) And rightfully so! First, you should know that all carbohydrate foods cause the body to release insulin into the blood. Insulin is a **storage** hormone, sometimes called an **anabolic** hormone. Insulin performs 3 roles in the body:
 1) Insulin helps drive sugar derived from carbohydrate foods into the muscles where it is stored as muscle glycogen. That's good as glycogen is the fuel tank for your bodybuilding workouts.
 2) Insulin also drives amino acids from the protein foods you eat into muscles to promote new muscle growth. That's advantageous as only amino acids from

protein can make new muscle tissue.

3) The final job is to stimulate body fat storage

Q) Now I'm really confused. How do I know if I am storing glycogen or body fat.
A) The first step in **inhibiting** body fat is to omit or avoid the things that cause #3/fat storage **and do the things that cause #1 and #2.**

Q) What causes #1 and #2...Glycogen storage and muscle growth?
A) Low to moderate blood insulin levels cause #1 and #2.

Q) What causes #3, fat storage?
A) Two things cause #3. Eating more carbs than your muscle glycogen tanks can handle. Remember, after glycogen tanks are full, all excess carbs will cause fat storage. The second factor that causes #3 is **high insulin levels.**

Q) How do I avoid high insulin levels?
A) By following these six steps. These things **lower** insulin level.

1) Divide your carbohydrate intake into 5 to 6 smaller meals. This forces you to control the total amount of carbohydrates you eat at one time. The more carbohydrates you eat at one sitting, the more insulin is released. For example, 2 bagels can release twice the amount of total insulin that one can release.

2) Eat fiber. Fiber, specifically **soluble** fibers found in oatmeal, fruits, and beans slow or "retard" the entry of sugar into the blood. When sugars from

carbohydrate foods enter the blood at a slower rate, less total insulin is released.

3) Eat vegetables. Vegetables contain insoluble fibers. Vegetables can help you stay lean because they are tremendously low in calories, so they can "replace" higher calorie carbohydrates. For example, instead of eating 2 cups of pasta, you can control calories, carbs, and insulin by cutting back to 1 1/2 cups of pasta but throw in a cup of mixed vegetables to "replace" the higher calorie pasta. Vegetables also make you feel full, like you have eaten a lot of food.

4) Eat protein with each meal. If you eat a bagel, alone, it may spike your insulin levels. If you eat a bagel with a small amount of chicken breast, the protein (and the small amount of fat found in the chicken) will "blunt" or modify insulin release. Proteins can alter the speed of sugar breakdown, so less insulin is released.

5) Include omega-3 fatty acids. Omega-3's are a special type of fat found in fish like salmon, mackeral, swordfish, tuna, blue fish or in supplementary capsules. Flax seed oil is non marine or vegetable source of omega-3 fatty acids. This fat can ultimately prevent high insulin release.

There are receptors for insulin on both fat cells and muscle cells. Fish oils make the receptors on muscle more sensitive to insulin. If muscles are **sensitive** to insulin, the body will not **output** a high level of insulin. Remember avoiding high insulin is important in controlling body fat and building muscle.

6) Avoid Saturated Fat. Saturated fat is the fat found in animal foods. The marbeling in pork, red

meat or the skin of chicken breast or the fat in the dark meat in both chicken breast and turkey contains saturated fat. Saturated fat works the exact opposite to fish oils. Saturated fat makes muscles **less sensitive** to the effects of insulin. When muscles tissue is less sensitive to insulin, the body responds by dumping *a whole lot* of insulin into the blood and high insulin is a "no-no" for the person hoping to stay lean.

Q) Does lowering insulin effect the appetite?
A) Yes, lower to moderate insulin levels are important to build muscle and store muscle glycogen. Controlling insulin also helps to control your appetite. High insulin can trigger your appetite.

Here's an easy example of how it works. Haven't you ever opened a box of cookies with the intent to eat just 1 or 2, yet you end up eating the entire box? Cookies are high in sugar, low in protein and they are completely lacking fiber so they break down into "blood sugar" with lightening speed which causes a big insulin burst. High insulin stimulates the appetite center in the brain **to eat more!** Plus, the job of insulin is **to clear excess sugar out of the blood.** High insulin, effectively clears too much sugar from the blood, leaving you with a "low blood sugar level." When blood sugar levels are low, **another** feedback message is sent to the brain. The message reads: "Warning! my sugar levels are low please eat some carbohydrates immediately to bring them back to normal!" You respond by eating more carbs to return sugar levels in the blood to normal levels. To summarize, excess insulin stimulates the appetite, then insulin removes sugar from the blood, which sets in motion the demand to eat even more! Control insulin levels to build muscle **and** to control both body fat levels as well as your appetite.

Q) How about protein. What is its role in bodybuilding nutrition?
A) Protein is the most important nutrient in bodybuilding nutrition. Protein makes muscles, period! If you do not eat the right amount of protein, you will not be able to build muscle.

Q) How much is enough?
A) You should eat at least one gram per pound of lean body weight or about a gram per pound of body weight. If you weigh 200, you need at least 200 grams a day. Some professional bodybuilders make better gains on 1.5 grams of protein per pound of body weight. Therefore a 200 pounder would eat 300 grams a day.

Q) I heard a gram per pound of bodyweight.
A) One gram of protein per pound of bodyweight is a very accurate ball park figure. However, one gram per pound of LBW is better because it takes into consideration "how much of you is really muscle." You could weigh 240 pounds, but your LBW may be only 190. Also, not everyone is the same. Although I believe one gram of protein per pound of LBW is best, you could require up to 1.5 grams of protein per pound of LBW which is quite a bit more.

Q) How does protein build muscle?
A) Muscle tissue is made of protein. When you train it effectively, you cause some micro damage to the tissue. In order for the tissue to heal and re-build itself, you have to take in more dietary protein.

Q) My friend is a nutritionist and he told me I do not need more protein to build, I need more carbs.
A) He's sort of right. You do need more carbohydrates as carbohydrates break down into sugar and sugar is the fuel source weight training muscles prefer to use. However, protein is the raw ingredients muscles need to repair, grow and make a bigger muscle. If you train hard and eat a low protein diet, you will not grow even if you stuff yourself with carbohydrates all day long! In fact, the opposite is true. If you fail to eat the right amount of protein and over stuff yourself with too many carbohydrates, your body will make a lot of fat with those carbohydrates and will have failed to grow due to a lack of "building" material in the form of dietary protein.

Q) I thought carbohydrates were "protein sparing."
A) They are. They spare your body from using protein as fuel - that's the definition of the word "protein sparing." Here's how protein sparing works...
    The fuel source for weight training is sugar. The sugar comes from carbo foods and is found in your blood. As you weight train, you use the sugar in the blood to power your training session and as the session progresses, the body stops using its "blood sugar" and begins to call upon muscle glycogen for additional sugar. When glycogen becomes low, the body starts to call on

yet another fuel source. That fuel source is protein. Protein is a "back-up" fuel source for sugar in weight training.

If you eat a low carbohydrate diet what do you think will happen? That's right, your body will quickly burn through its glycogen tanks and look for protein as a fuel. By eating **sufficient** carbohydrates, you are effectively causing a "protein sparing" effect. That is, you use carbs for fuel - not protein.

Q) I thought "protein sparing" meant carbohydrates build muscle.
A) No. It means exactly how it sounds ...spares the body from using its protein.

Q) What happens if the body uses protein for fuel during weight training?
A) You lose muscle!

Q) How so?
A) Muscles are made of protein. If you do not eat sufficient amounts of carbohydrates and your body starts to use protein as a back up fuel source, the body tears down its own muscle tissue to obtain protein as fuel. You've heard of a car "running on fumes?" Well, a lack of carbohydrates forces your body to do the same thing - it rips its muscle apart - so you can continue to do your weight training workout.

Q) Can't I eat more protein to prevent that from happening?
A) Yes, eating more protein can help. If your body calls upon protein as fuel and you have a bunch in the blood from a previous meal, your muscles can use

some of the dietary protein as fuel rather than tear down and use muscle protein. However, the best approach is to eat the right amount of carbohydrates to provide the fuel to train and the right amount of protein to build muscle.

Q) Doesn't insulin build muscle - you said it was an "anabolic" hormone.
A) You are right. Insulin is considered an anabolic hormone. Insulin **allows** amino acids from protein foods to get **into** muscle. So, in that way, your nutritionist is accurate. If you don't have carbohydrates, you don't have an insulin release which makes it very difficult for amino acids from protein to get into muscle to cause growth. Ultimately, protein is most important as ***insulin can not build muscle without protein.***

Q) How else is protein important?
A) Protein is required to make new enzymes and hormones in the body. There are millions of enzymes in the body that support muscle growth and we know the hormones called testosterone, insulin, growth hormone, and thyroid hormone all effect muscle building in one way or another. Failing to eat enough protein will inhibit optimal muscle growth as protein is necessary to make enzymes and hormones.

Q) How many total calories do I need in a day?
A) The answer depends on whether your goal is to lose fat or to add muscle mass.

Shedding fat requires that you eat less energy in the form of calories each day. Building muscle requires you increase your total caloric intake.

Q) How do I get started?
A) There is only one right way to start. Add up all the calories you eat in 7 days and divide the grand total by 7. This will provide you with a "picture" or your diet. The answer you get will tell you, on average, how many calories you typically eat each day. For example, you may eat a sporadic diet. One day you may eat 3000 calories, another day you might eat only 2200 calories and on a third, you may eat 2700 calories and so on. What is important is to find your **average daily caloric intake.**

Q) After establishing my average daily caloric intake, what should I do next?
A) To lose fat, you should reduce calories. To add muscle, you must increase calories.

Q) What about those tables that will tell me how many calories I should eat each day depending on my activity level.
A) They don't work. Your current average daily caloric intake exerts the **most important and greatest bearing** on where to start your nutritional strategy.

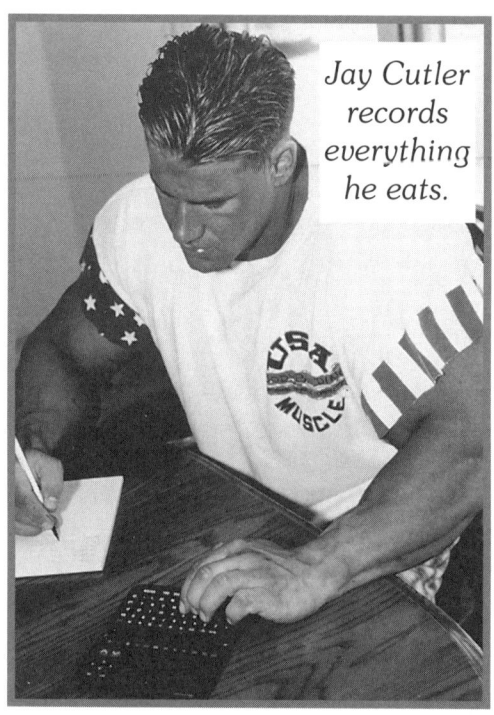

Jay Cutler records everything he eats.

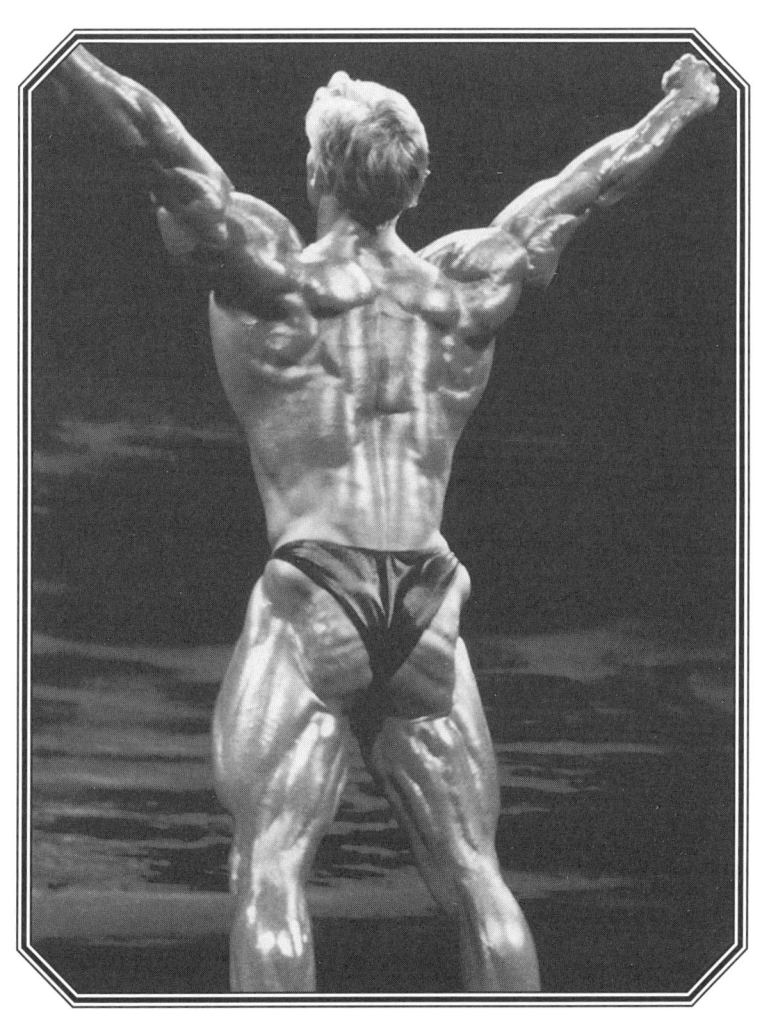

North American Champ, Dave Fischer attains incredibly low body fat levels with an adequate protein intake.

QUESTIONS DEALING WITH ADDING MASS

Q) I want to add mass, what do I do after finding my average daily caloric intake?

A) Adding mass depends on two important nutritional factors. You must eat sufficient protein to build new muscle and you must increase your calories. Additional calories will provide you with the fuel to train hard to stimulate muscle growth and, recovery and repair is a energy dependent process.

Q) What do you mean by energy dependent?

A) In order for new muscle to be built, the body needs more fuel. If you train hard and do not take in enough calories, the rebuilding and growth process will be short circuited, and new muscle will not be built!

Q) How many additional calories do I need above my average daily caloric intake?

A) Here is where you must be careful. Increasing your calories too high can increase body fat stores. Therefore, I suggest you increase your calories by 20%. That is, you must eat 20% more calories than you average daily caloric intake.

For example, if you are eating 3000 calories a day, increasing your calories by 20% would mean eating another 600 calories daily. Your **new daily caloric intake** should be no more than 3600 calories. Eating 3700, and above may cause you to add unwanted body fat.

After increasing calories, you should strive to eat 6 meals a day. If you have a hard time staying lean, you may have to take drastic measures and spread your food intake into 8 meals!

Q) Why so many meals?
A) The trick in adding fat free muscle mass is to get as much nutrition into your body without eating an abundance of calories a one sitting. Of course, you must stay within the parameters of your caloric requirements. Therefore, the person eating 3600 calories should avoid overloading his body with too much calories, food and nutrients all at once. This can only be achieved with 6 small meals a day.

Q) What if I can not eat 6 times a day?
A) You can not increase your muscle mass without adding body fat on 3 or even 4 meals a day unless you have a race-horse metabolism, fabulous genetics, or a combination of the two.

Q) What kinds of calories should I eat?
A) While increasing your total calories is pertinent in adding fat free muscle mass, your results and progress are strongly correlated with your protein intake. If you eat the right amount of calories, but the wrong amount of protein, you will not be successful in adding muscle weight. In fact, if you increase your calories and eat too little protein, it is possible to add mostly body fat!

Q) What is the right amount of protein?
A) Building mass requires you eat roughly one gram of protein per pound of bodyweight. Some will have to increase their protein intake to a higher level - to 1.5 grams of protein for each pound of bodyweight.

Q) How about carbs and fat?
A) Let's address fat first. Fat is essential to your body. You require it in small amounts each day. Specifically, the human body requires only 1% of all its calories from essential fat. Essential fats are found in vegetable oils.

These fats make hormone like substances called prostaglandins which may help assist in some physiological properties that may be beneficial to the bodybuilder. These properties include increase blood flow to muscle tissue, an anti-inflammatory effect sore muscles and they support the immune system and the production of growth hormone and testosterone.

Q) How much fat do I need?
A) The bodybuilder seeking mass should limit his caloric intake to 15% dietary fat. This can be easily obtained. Most of it (the 15% fat) will be obtained from eating your protein food. **All** protein foods contain fat and fat is found in small amounts in all of your carbohydrate foods. Dietary fat from oils can be obtained from PAM to coat cooking skillets and from using lo-fat salad dressings.

It is totally absurd to increase your fat intake in hopes of adding new muscle. Diets that are high in fat will not help you build muscle. High fat diets **are low carbohydrate diets.** Carbohydrates are the first and best fuel source for weight training and they release insulin which assists in "getting" amino acids from protein foods into your muscles to make bigger and new muscle tissue. Increasing your fat forces you to decrease your carbohydrates. Recall a low carbohydrate intake will force our body to use muscle tissue as fuel!

Q) What about carbs? How many do I need?
A) I'll get to that. First let's build your diet based on 3600 calories step by step.

The least important nutrient that effects muscle growth is dietary fat. Limit your fat to 15% of your total calories

This amount of fat is naturally occurring in your protein foods. A diet that is low in fat, one that includes lean sources of protein like chicken and turkey breast, egg whites, a moderate amount of whole eggs, and lean meat will provide 15% dietary fat.

To find your fat calories, multiply 15% by your **new average daily caloric intake.**

Example: 3600 x .15 = 540 calories of fat is naturally occurring in the food you eat.

Q) How many grams of fat is 540 calories of fat.
A) One gram of fat yields 9 calories in the body. To find the amount of grams of fat you can eat each day, **divide your fat calories by 9.**

Example: 540/9 = 60 grams of fat.

Again, this fat will automatically "show up" in your diet as it is found in the protein foods you eat and to a lesser degree, in your carbohydrate foods. It's not important to count your fat. Simply eat lean protein sources and do not add oils and butter to your foods.

Q) After I establish the fat I should eat, what do I do next.

A) Subtract the fat calories from your **new** average daily caloric intake. The remaining calories will be divided into appropriate amounts of protein and carbohydrates.

Example: 3600 - 540 = 3060 calories.
3060 calories will be divided into proteins and carbs.

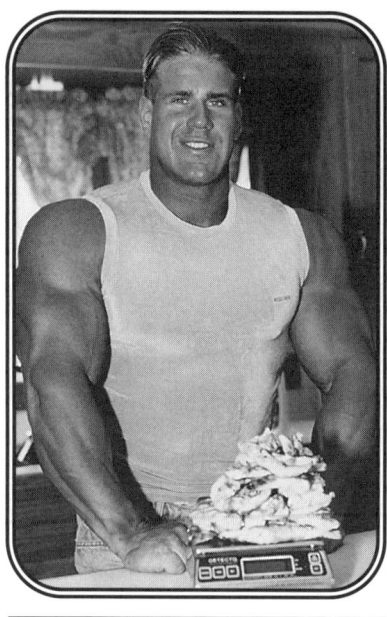

Jay always meets his daily protein requirement.

SPEED BUMP

Fat is the least important nutrient in muscle building. Your body needs protein to build muscle and carbohydrates to train hard and to help get protein in muscles.

Q) How much of the 3060 calories should be protein and how much should be carbohydrates?
A) You need 1 to 1.5 grams of protein per pound of bodyweight to grow. You also must know a nutritional

fact about protein.
One gram of protein yields 4 calories in the body. To find your protein requirements, multiply your body weight by 1.

Example: Bodyweight x 1 = daily protein requirements
: 200 x 1 = 200 grams of protein daily

To find carbohydrates, you must subtract your protein **calories** from 3060. The remaining number will be allotted to carbohydrates.

Example 200 grams protein x 4 calories = 800 calories of protein.

3060-800 = 2260 calories remaining to be allotted to carbohydrate foods.

Q) How do I find the amount of grams of carbohydrates to eat?
A) Follow this nutritional fact.
Each gram of carbohydrates yields 4 calories
To find your carbohydrates in grams, divide 2260 by 4.
Example 2260/4 = 565 grams of carbohydrates

STOP! (review pages 96-103)

The important numbers are these. The 200 pound bodybuilder in the example above who eats, on average, 3000 calories a day, should increase his caloric consumption (by 20%) to 3600 calories a day with 565 grams of carbohydrates and 200 grams of protein.

SPEED BUMP

Individualize your diet by following the flow chart. This is the summary of the previous questions.

Step 1 Find your **average daily caloric intake (ADCI).** Add up all the calories you eat in 7 days. Divide by 7. This is your average daily caloric intake.

Step 2 To add mass, increase calories. Most can add muscle without body fat by increasing their ADCI by 20%. Multiply your **ADCI** in step one by 20%. Add the answer to the number in step 1. **This is your new average daily caloric intake.**

Step 3 Find the fat calories. Low fat diets provide 15% fat. Multiply your **new** ADCI in step 2 by .15.

Step 4 Subtract the fat calories in step 3 from the **new** ADCI found in step 2.

Step 5 To find protein requirements, multiply your bodyweight by 1.

Step 6 To find protein calories, multiply the answer to step 5 by 4. (Protein requirement x 4.)

Step 7 Subtract the answer to step 6 from the answer to step 4.

Step 8 To find carbohydrates in grams, divide the answer in step 7 by 4.

Q) What will happen if I *increase* my caloric intake by more than 20% **above** my ADCI?

A) You will add body fat along with muscle tissue. If you are worried about adding body fat, you can increase your calories by a smaller number. Try 10% or 15% above your ADCI.

Q) What about ratios. I heard you should eat a diet that is 65% carbohydrates, 25% protein and 10% dietary fat.

A) The ratio of 65/25/10 is simply a "ball park" recommendation. However, the problem is you become a slave to the ratio. A **custom** approach to a mass gain strategy requires you find *your own* average daily caloric intake and to base your entire program on *your own* personal protein requirements.

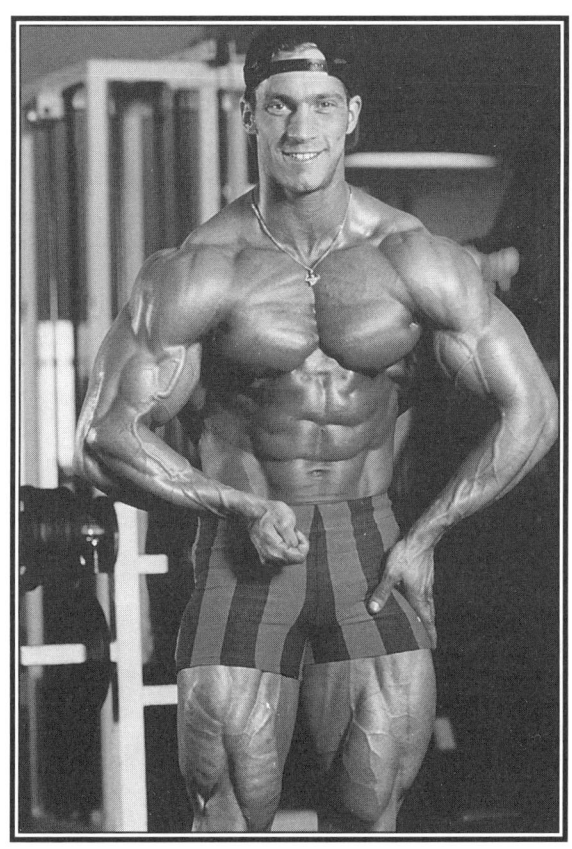

*Canadian Champ, Remi Zuri
ate 5 meals a day to build his awesome physique.*

Q) Besides being a **customized plan,** what else makes the mass plan different?
A) The grams of carbohydrates you find following this method is, generally, the **maximum** amount of carbs you can consume on a mass gaining plan without storing body fat. Your own carbohydrate number in grams (as found in step 8) is the amount of carbs it takes to "fill" and saturate your muscles and liver with glycogen. Any additional carbs will "spill over" and store as body fat.

Q) What if I choose 1.5 grams of protein per pound of bodyweight to find my protein requirements.
A) No problem. It's true, there is some individuality in nutrition. If you choose to eat a higher protein diet, you still follow the same flow chart (page 104). Your final answers will be somewhat different in that a higher protein intake will force you to consume fewer carbohydrates. In the example I put together, the 200 pounder who eats 3600 calories, 565 grams of carbs and 200 grams of protein would alter his carbohydrate intake to 465 grams of carbohydrates and 300 grams of protein by following the exact same 8 steps.

Q) What about meal timing?
A) Adding mass without adding body fat can not be achieved by simply establishing a new average daily caloric intake and eating the right amounts of carbohydrates and protein. You **must** break your meals into 6 smaller ones to maximize the absorption of your food and nutrition and to prevent "stuffing" yourself at one sitting.

The body can not store protein to any large degree, so it is best to divide your protein intake into 6 **equal size servings.** This will give your body a constant flow of amino acids from protein to build and repair new tissue.

Dividing up your carbohydrates is also important to cause muscle growth and to prevent and inhibit fat storage. Remember, carbohydrates release insulin which increases protein entry into muscles. The bottom line here is simple, eat your carbs and protein together. No carbs = no growth.

Dividing up your carbohydrate intake also helps to "manage" insulin. Recall too much insulin from eating too many carbs at one time can cause fat storage. Altering your carbohydrate intake will prevent you from eating too much at once.

Q) How should I divide up my carbohydrates.
A) Eat more at two times during the day. Eat 25% of your carbs after training and 20 to 25% in the morning at your first meal.

Q) Why eat 25% of my carbs after training?
A) You have to eat more of your carbs after training to "re-pay" the carbs you used up during your weight training session. Also, a higher carb intake will "spike" insulin levels after training. High insulin levels at this time are ideal as they "force" the extra carbohydrates you are eating into the muscles to make new muscle glycogen. Furthermore, high insulin after training, helps to facilitate amino acids into the muscles for growth and repair.

Q) If high insulin is so good, why don't I always keeps my insulin levels super elevated with more and more carbohydrates?
A) Because a high insulin level **at rest** causes fat storage. Furthermore, too many carbs equates to too many total calories which promotes body fat storage. Remember, you have to eat **according to your own personal average daily caloric intake.** The number you find in step 8 is, roughly, your maximum daily carbohydrate allotment. It's the amount of carbs you can eat without storing fat.

Q) Why eat more carbs in my first meal?
A) Blood sugar and glycogen levels are low in the morning. If you eat more carbs at your first meal of the day, your body must restore muscle glycogen and bring blood sugar levels up first.

Q) So, I can eat simple carbs after training?
A) Yes.

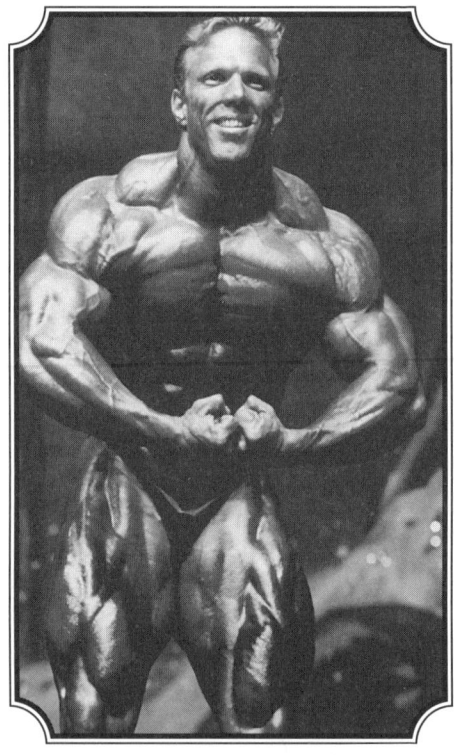

Dave Fischer doesn't fear simple carbs – as long as they fall into his post training meal.

Q) If I eat 25% of my total carbohydrate intake after I train, how many of those should be simple carbs?

A) First, let me recap and make it perfectly clear. Your post training meal is the most important of all your meals each day. Eating the ideal amount of carbs after you train can transform a catabolic (muscle wasting) state into an anabolic (growth!) state in a flash. The success of your meal depends on the **total amount** of post training carbs you eat **and** on how many complex to simple carbs you eat.

Eating sufficient carbs will

a) re-store muscle glycogen and

b) deliver amino acids from the protein you eat into recovering muscles. Post training carbohydrates also counter-balances the release of a muscle wasting hormone called cortisol. Recall from previous training questions, training sessions that last too long, volumous training sessions and low muscle glycogen stores cause the release of cortisol which causes muscles to be torn down-to be used as fuel.

The manipulation of carbs to promote growth is simple. First, multiply your total carbo intake by 25%. Follow the example below...

Total carb intake = 400 grams

Post training carb intake should be 25% of the total carb intake.

400 x .25 = 100 grams of carbs should be eaten after training.

Q) Ok, but what amount of the 100 carbs should be simple carbs?

A) An approximate ratio of complex to simple carbs is

3:1. Eat 3 times as much complex carbs compared to simple carbs. For example, the bodybuilder who eats 100 grams of carbs after training should eat 75 grams of complex carbs and 25 grams of simple carbs. Here is a simple chart that includes 3 categories.

PTCI stands for "post training carbohydrate intake"
CC stands for "complex carbohydrate intake" (in grams)
SC stands for "simple carbohydrate intake" (in grams)

PTCI	CC	SC
50	38 1 ounce hot cereal 2 slices wheat bread 6 ounce yam	12 1/2 cup applesauce 1 tablespoon jam 1 tablespoon raisins
100	76 3 ounces hot cereal 4 slices wheat bread 12 ounce yam	24 1/2 cup applesauce 2 tablespoons jam 2 tablespoons raisins
150	113 4 ounces hot cereal 6 slices wheat bread 18 ounce yam	37 3/4 cup applesauce 3 tablespoons jam 3 tablespoon raisins

Q) If I eat 100 grams of carbs at breakfast and another 100 grams after training, I will have 200 carbs remaining out of my 400 gram total for the day. How many carbs should I eat at my remaining 4 meals?
A) Simply divide 200 by the 4 remaining meals, for 50 grams of carbs per meal.

Q) I have found my own numbers for total calories, carbs and protein. How do I know how much of each food to eat at each meal?
A) Refer to the chart on page 111. Simply plug in

your numbers. Here are common lean sources of protein and their approximate protein and fat content in grams. All are virtually fat free in carbohydrates.

FOOD	PROTEIN (grams)	FAT (grams)
4 ounces chicken breast, pcw	18	3
4 ounces turkey breast, pcw	30	2
4 ounces cod fish, pcw	20	1
4 ounces haddock, pcw	19	1
4 ounces salmon, pcw	20	10
4 ounces swordfish, pcw	21	7
6 ounce can tuna	30	5
4 ounces round steak, pcw	27	5
4 ounces flank steak, pcw	24	7
2 eggs, large	12	12
6 egg whites	18	0
1/3 cup American Bodybuilding Superior Whey Protein Powder	24	2

These Carbohydrate foods yield approximately 23 to 25 grams of carbohydrates. All are virtually fat free and contain less than 2 grams of protein.

4 ounce potato, pcw	1/2 cup canned corn
3 ounce yam, pcw	1 pear, apple, banana, large
3/4 cup cooked rice	
1 ounce pasta, pcw	10 ounces orange juice
1 ounce hot cereal, pcw	2 Fig Newton Cookies
1 slice whole grain bread	1/4 cup Grape Nuts Cereal
1/2 bagel	1 cup each: Cheerios, Corn Flakes
1 english muffin	

*pcw = "pre-cooked weight"

** Vegetables such as beets, broccoli, carrots, cauliflower, celery, cucumbers, lettuce, spinach, onions and peppers provide very few calories in the form of carbohydrates. However, they are an important source of fiber, vitamins and minerals and should be included in at least 3 of your 6 daily meals.

Q) What if I want to take my mass gaining diet to the extreme and eat 8 to 10 meals a day?
A) In theory, 8 to 10 meals a day may be better than 5 and 6 as more meals should **really** maximize nutrient absorption. If you choose to take such a novel approach, **let your schedule dictate the number of meals you eat.** If you wake up very early and go to bed late, you can eat 10 times. However, if you wake up later and go to bed earlier, you probably can fit fewer meals into your day - perhaps 8. Either way, to "fit" that many feedings into your schedule, you will have to eat every 1 1/2 to 2 hours.

Q) How do I find the amount of calories, carbs and protein to eat?
A) Use the "8 step" method on page 104. Then, simply divide your total carb intake by the number of meals you plan to eat. Also, divide your total protein intake by the number of meals you plan to eat.

For example if you require 200 grams of protein a day and 500 grams of carbohydrates, simply divide these total by 8 or ten meals.

200 grams of protein split evenly into 8 meals yields 25 grams of protein at each meal.

200 grams of protein split evenly into 10 meals

yields 20 grams of protein at each meal.

500 grams of carbohydrates split evenly into 8 meals yields approximately 62 grams of carbs at each meal.

500 grams of carbohydrates split evenly into 10 meals yields approximately 50 grams of carbs at each meal.

Q) What about breakfast and the post training meal?
A) If you are eating 8, 9 or 10 times a day, there is no need to eat a greater amount of your carbs at these two times as your body is **truly constantly being exposed to a non stop slow flow of amino acids and sugar** which, in research papers, can totally offset muscle breakdown and, in theory, can maximize muscle glycogen synthesis without having to alter your carb intake in the morning or after training.

FAT LOSS QUESTIONS

Q) My goal is to lose fat. Where do I start?

A) Let me correct you. Your goal is to lose fat **and retain your muscle mass.** Holding onto muscle is the **most** important aspect in altering your appearance while dieting. Most who embark on a fat loss program lose muscle along with body fat.

To lose fat, you must eat less calories and exercise aerobically to use up body fat stores. The procedure to get started is very similar to the "8 step" program found on page 102 - 103. However, after finding your average daily caloric intake, you must **reduce** your caloric intake to create a deficit.

Here is the 8 step Program for fat loss

Step 1 Find your **average daily caloric intake (ADCI).** Add up all the calories you eat in 7 days. Divide by 7. This is your average daily caloric intake.

Step 2 To lose fat, decrease calories. Cut your caloric intake by 10, 15 or 20% maximum. Multiply your **ADCI** in step 1 by 15% (or 10% or 20%). Subtract the answer from the ADCI in step 1. **This is your new average daily caloric intake.**

Step 3 Find the fat calories. Low fat diets provide 15% fat. Multiply the **new** ADCI in step 2 by .15.

Step 4 Subtract the fat calories in step 3 from the **new** ADCI in step 2.

Step 5 To find protein requirements, multiply your bodyweight by 1.

Step 6 To find protein calories, multiply the answer in step 5 by 4. (Protein requirement x 4.)

Step 7 Subtract the answer to step 6 from the answer to step 4.

Step 8 To find carbohydrates in grams, divide the answer in step 7 by 4.

Q) What will happen if I **reduce** my calories by more than 20% **below** the ADCI?
A) You will lose muscle tissue along with body fat. When you lose muscle, your metabolism slows which, in turn, makes fat loss very difficult.

Q) Should I eat 25% of my carbs at breakfast and another 25% after training like the person seeking mass gains.
A) Absolutely. These are the two times dieting muscles need an insulin spike to "turn on" anabolism, the "switch" that allows the dieting bodybuilder to retain muscle! You should, like the mass seeking bodybuilder, eat 6 meals a day as well.

Q) I have found my own numbers for total calories, carbs and protein. How do I know how much of each food to eat at each meal?
A) Refer to the chart on page 111. Simply plug in your numbers.

Example of 8 Step Fat Loss Method
Step 1   21,000 total calories in 7 days
         Divide by 7 = 3000 calories ADCI
Step 2   3000 ADCI
          20% reduction from ADCI
          600

         3000 ADCI
         - 600 caloric reduction
         2400 calories, new ADCI

Step 3   2400 ADCI
          15% fat (successful diets yield 15% fat)
          360 fat calories
Step 4   2400 new ADCI
         - 360 fat calories
          2040 calories to be allotted to protein and carbs.
Step 5   Bodyweight = 150 pounds
          150 x 1 = 150 grams of protein
Step 6   150 x 4 = 600 calories of protein
Step 7   2040 answer to Step 4
         - 600
          1440 calories remain
Step 8   1440 ÷ 4 = 360 grams of carbohydrates

The final numbers are: 2400 calories
                         150 grams protein
                         360 grams carbs

Daily Example
Protein: 150 ÷ 6 meals = 25 grams per meal
Carbs: 25% of (360) = 90 grams at breakfast
           25% of (360) = 90 grams after train
           180 remaining = (Divide by 4 meals)
              45 grams per meal

Meal 1	25 grams protein	90 grams carbs
Meal 2	25 grams protein	45 grams carbs
Meal 3	25 grams protein	45 grams carbs
Meal 4	25 grams protein	45 grams carbs
	Train here	Train here
Meal 5	25 grams protein	90 grams carbs
Meal 6	25 grams protein	45 grams carbs

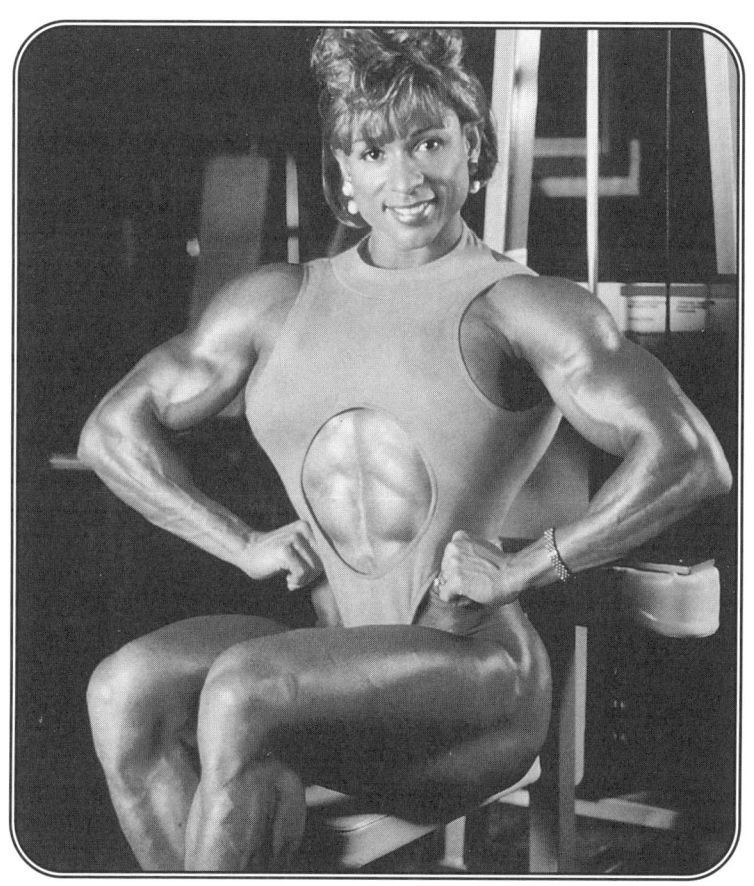

Laura relies on cardio only to burn fat – never to build muscle!

Q) How much fat can I expect to lose?
A) First, understand to lose fat one pound of fat one of 3 scenarios must occur

   a) you must subtract 3500 calories from your diet over a 7 to 10 day period

   b) you must expend 3500 calories via exercise over a 7 to 10 day period

   c) you must combine a and b and subtract and expend a total of 3500 calories over a 7 to 10 day period. The time it takes to lose a pound of fat will vary from person to person. Follow the graph below to guestimate the length of time it will take you to lose a pound of fat **with a reduction in calories.**

ADCI	10% RD	15% RD	20% RD	Approximate time to lose 1 pound body fat (3500 divided by figure in RD)
3000	300	450	600	3500/300 = 11 days 3500/450 = 8 days 3500/600 = 6 days
2200	220	330	440	3500/220 = 16 days 3500/330 = 11 days 3500/440 = 8 days

ADCI= "average daily caloric intake"
10% RD = 10 percent reduction *from* the ADCI
15% RD = 15 percent reduction *from* the ADCI
20% RD = 20 percent reduction *from* the ADCI

Q) How about if I do aerobic work?
A) Remember, you must either omit 3500 calories from your diet over a 7 to 10 day period to lose a pound of fat or you can expend, through exercise, 3500 calories from your diet over the same time frame.

A popular approach is to include aerobic exercise with a calorie reduced diet to cause fat loss. Generally, aerobic exercise burns about 10 calories each minute. So, a thirty minute session should use up 300 calories of stored body fat.

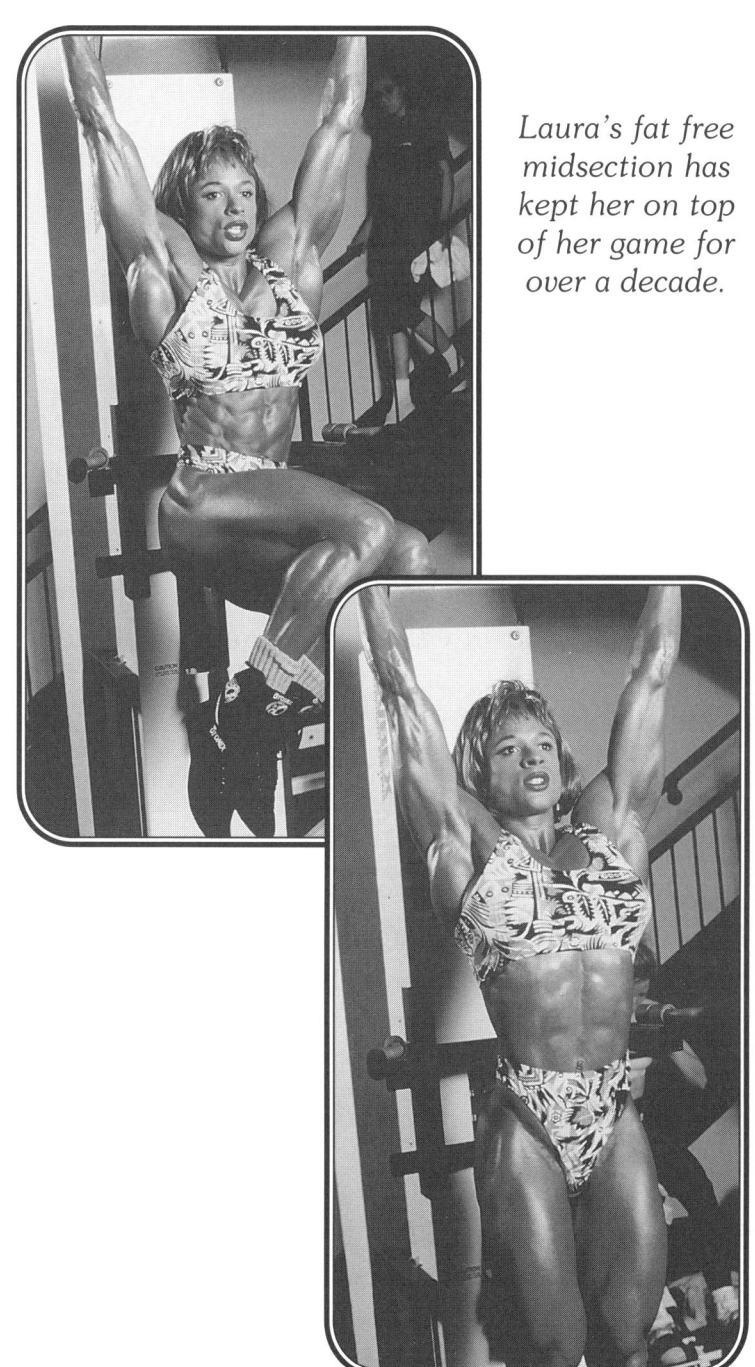

Laura's fat free midsection has kept her on top of her game for over a decade.

If you choose to combine aerobic exercise and a calorie reduced diet, simply divide 3500 calories by 2. (3500/2 = 1750)

To lose a pound of fat you must reduce your calories by 1750 over 7 days and increase your caloric expenditure by 1750 over 7 days.

To shed 1750 calories from your diet, you must cut 250 calories out of your daily caloric intake (1750/7 = 250)

To burn off 250 calories from your fat stores, you must expend 250 calories a day through your aerobic sessions. (1750/7 = 250)

Q) Does all aerobic activity burn 10 calories a minute? How can a minute of walking compare to a minute of jogging?
A) Your right, in **general,** you must perform your aerobic work in your "target heart rate."

Q) What is "target heart rate"
A) Target heart rate measures your level of aerobic exercise intensity. The "target range" can be found by finding your maximum heart rate - the approximate maximum amount of heart beats your heart can beat in one minute during (maximal) aerobic exercise. Your maximum heart rate can be estimated by subtracting your age from 220.

For example, a 20 year old would have a maximum heart rate of 200 beats during one minute of all out-prolonged aerobic exercise.

The target heart rate is a percentage of one's maximum. The target heart rate is defined as anywhere between 60% and 75% of the maximum heart rate.

Follow the easy chart below to find your target heart rate.

HEART RATE AT AGE...	60%	65%	70%	75%
20	120	130	140	150
25	117	127	137	146
30	114	124	133	143
35	111	120	130	139
40	108	117	126	135
45	105	114	122	131
50	102	110	119	127
55	99	107	115	123
60	96	104	111	119
65	93	101	108	115

Q) Which intensity is best for me?
A) In general, choose the higher levels, closer to 70 or 75% because the harder you work, the more total calories you burn.

However, if you are just starting an aerobic program, choose 60% As that level of intensity becomes less stressful and easier to maintain, you can gradually progress to 65% then 70% and up to 75%

Q) Does it matter what time I do my exercise.
A) Yes. Aerobics performed in the morning, on an empty stomach will allow you to more readily "tap" into stored body fat as fuel.

Q) Why?

A) Recall the fuel for aerobics is fat. This fat is derived from dietary fat (the fat you eat in your food) or from stored body fat. If you eat a meal within a couple of hours of performing your aerobic exercise, some of the fuel used during exercise will come from the fat in your food and some from your stored fat. Furthermore, recall that carbohydrate foods cause a release in the hormone called insulin. Insulin is a **storage hormone.** It causes muscle cells and fat cells to uptake and store sugar or fat. Besides **storing** fuels, it can **prevent** fat cell breakdown. Abstaining from all food before your aerobic session will allow you to more readily tap stored body fat as fuel.

Index of Common Bodybuilding Terms

—A—

ACETALDEHYDE in an end product along with carbon dioxide during alcohol fermentation. This enzyme (acetaldehyde) is found in organisms like yeast.

ACETIC ACID is an end product of the anaerobic breakdown of glucose.

ACETYL CO ENZYME A is an energy intermediate that is stimulated from eating above and beyond basal caloric needs. It is required to form body fat from carbohydrates and dietary fat. Many bodybuilders use the supplement carcinia gambogia which can temporarily inhibit the formation of acetyl co enzyme A. Suppressing the formation of acetyl co enzyme A can prevent the storage of body fat.

ACETYLCHOLINE is a neurotransmitter that is released from the nerve ending and binds with cholinergic nicotinic receptors which are special receptor cites located on the surface of the muscle cell. This process causes the contraction of that muscle.

ACIDOPHILUS is also known as "lactobacillus acidophilus", a friendly bacteria found in yogurt. Acidophilus is also found in the human digestive tract. It helps digestion and fights yeast infections in women. It has also been shown to strengthen and support the immune system.

ADP see ATP.

ADRENAL GLANDS are located on top of the kidneys. There are two parts the adrenal medulla and the adrenal cortex. The medulla releases epinephrine and norepinephrine in response to hard workouts. Epinephrine and epinephrine increase cardiac output, (the heart's contraction) and cause the body to break down fatty acids and glycogen (into sugar) for fuel. The cortex releases cortisol and aldosterone in response to hard workouts. Cortisol breaks down fat for fuel but also tears down muscle tissue. Aldosterone causes water and sodium retention.

ADRENALIN is a stress hormone that is released when the body experiences stress, either physical, like when preparing for a big dead lift, or mental, when someone tells you your best friends was just in a car accident. The sympathetic nervous system releases two neurotransmitters in the brain called epinephrine and norepinephrine (NE). They increase the heart rate, and cause blood vessels to dilate to improve blood flow. They trigger the fat cell to release fatty acids as fuel while sparing the use of glucose for fuel. Bodybuilders use ephedrine and Ma Huang to release the very same neurotransmitters. They hope to increase fat breakdown. NE also increases body temperature so more calories are burned as heat rather than stored or used to make ATP.

ADRENOCORTICAL HORMONE (ACTH) is a polypeptide ("Protein hormone) hormone that is made, stored and released by the anterior pituitary gland in response to stress. ACTH stimulates the production and release of cortisol by the adrenal cortex. Cortisol acts to increase sugar levels in the blood by breaking down amino acids to make glucose. (Some of these aminos come from muscle mass; the result is muscle loss.)

ALACTACID MECHANISM refers to the metabolism of glucose in the body. Glucose is broken down into pyruvic acid and lactic acid is also formed during strenuous workouts. Lactic acid can seep out of the muscle and into the blood. Here it inhibits (prevents) muscle contraction. However, when exercise intensity drops, lactic acid can be resynthesized into pyruvic acid to be used as fuel.

ALANINE is an amino acid that is released from the muscle into the blood when carbohydrate stores in the muscle run low. Alanine is sent to the liver where it is converted into glucose. This glucose is sent back into the blood stream where it is used as fuel and it spares the release of further alanine from the muscle. The process of alanine release from muscle tissue is a catabolic event; the opposite of the desired anabolic state referenced below. Eating sufficient carbohydrates will suppress this catabolic process. Red meat is also high in alanine. Those who eat red meat may use the alanine from the food to make glucose if the body demands so, due to a lowered carbohydrate intake.

ALBUMIN is a protein carrier found in the blood. There are lots of things floating around in the blood stream that can not bee seen with the naked eye. One of these is albumin; other things include gasses like oxygen, nitrogen, and carbon dioxide, minerals, and waste products like urea.
    Albumin is a plasma (blood) protein and is produced in the liver. It serves as a carrier for thyroxin and calcium in the blood and regulates the pressure in the bloodstream. When the amount of protein in the blood falls too low, the liver reacts by making more albumin.

ALCOHOL is unique because it is both a drug and a

food. It is also unique because it can be both beneficial to the health as well as detrimental. Alcohol, specifically red wine, contains tanins and antioxidants derived from the grapes that have been shown to fight bacteria and free radicals. Alcohol in moderation, the equivalent to 12 ounces of wine daily has been shown to lower total cholesterol levels, to increase HDL levels, and to dilate the vascular system. Such dilation acts as a "toner" to keep the veins strong and flexible. Alcohol can act as a mild thermogenic agent as well. Six ounces of wine can speed up the metabolism. Alcohol directly stimulates the liver. Apparently, this stimulation will cause the body to burn more calories. Ironically, more alcohol will over tax the liver and slow the metabolic rate.

Alcohol strips the body of folic acid and many B vitamins. It also must be cleared through the liver before it enters the blood. Continuous and excess alcohol consumption can permanently damage the liver.

Bodybuilders sometimes drink alcohol the final two days before a show when cutting back on fluid intake. When the body is deprived of fluids, it releases ADH or anti-diuretic hormone to conserve or hold water in the body. Alcohol interferes with this hormone release, so the body can not hold and conserve water. Alcohol in itself is a diuretic. It rids the body of water but the body can not react and fight back by holding water since alcohol also interferes with ADH release.

ALDOSTERONE is a salt retaining hormone released by the adrenal cortex which covers the tip of the kidney. Aldosterone increases the reabsorption of sodium. When a high salt diet is consumed the body releases less aldosterone, so it (sodium) can be passed through the body and excreted. When sodium is restricted, the body releases more aldosterone to retain sodium. Aldosterone is also affected by blood potassium levels. When potassium is high, the body will release more aldosterone to retain sodium for a favorable potassium to sodium balance. Drinking excess amounts of water can also trigger aldosterone release. Too much water will cause the body to pump out large amounts of sodium. If lots of water is consumed coupled with a salt restricted diet, the body will output more aldosterone in an attempt to hold sodium.

Bodybuilders who use ephedrine before going on state to compete should know that it stimulates the sympathetic nervous system which slows the blood flow to the kidneys. Decreasing blood flow to the kidneys causes the body to output more aldosterone and therefore water retention could be a problem.

ALFALFA is a natural diuretic and a source of octacosanol.

ALPHA KETOGLUTARATE is the keto acid of the important amino acid called glutamine. When a bodybuilder trains hard, he puts himself under a lot of stress which over burdens the immune system. The immune system uses glutamine as a fuel. This glutamine is derived from muscles. Muscles give up glutamine to improve and support immunity, but low muscle glutamine levels are associated with a lack of muscle growth and a lack in recovery. To offset this, bodybuilders can use alpha ketoglutarate. It supplies glutamine to the muscles without adding ammonia. Ammonia is a toxic by product that is present in protein metabolism and protein breakdown. Ammonia interferes with ATP production. The branched chain amino acids are also good at preserving glutamine, but they produce ammonia.

ALPHA-KETOGLUTARATE is an intermediary in the krebs cycle. It acts as an ammonia scavenger (lowers the amount of ammonia in the body). Ammonia is produced with a high protein diet or with hard weight training sessions. It can prevent muscle contraction. Alpha ketoglutarate is also related to glutamine. It is an ammonia free carbon form of glutamine. In supplemental form it can have the beneficial effects of glutamine without the ammonia build up that glutamine can produce (all amino acids produce ammonia).

AMINO ACIDS are the building blocks of the protein foods we eat. Building muscle requires the eight essential amino acids that are found in all animal source proteins including milk and eggs, fish, turkey, chicken, and beef. These eight can not be produced by the body, so we must consume them each day. Taking individual amino acids in supplemental form has no net effect on muscle growth. However, the branched chain amino acids can be used directly by the muscle as fuel and spare muscle breakdown during work or when calories are reduced. The best way to get amino acids for bodybuilding is from foods or from low-heat whey protein powders. Since the body can not store amino acids to any significant degree, the bodybuilder should eat five smaller meals a day to keep a constant level of amino acids in the blood.

AMPHETAMINES are drugs that mimic adrenalin in the body. Using these drugs, one can work more, and sleep less. However, in time, the body will experience a "crash" where it becomes impossible to function without the drug because the body's own hormone that amphetamines mimic (adrenalin) becomes severely depleted. Even getting out of bed can become impossible. Abusing these drugs can cause long term memory loss, and can over tax the adrenal glands, the location where adrenalin is naturally formed. Once this occurs, permanent kidney damage can result.

Dieters have used these over the years to suppress appetite.

AMYLASE is a digestive enzyme located in the salivary glands and pancreas. It is secreted in the mouth and in the small intestines to break down starches (polysaccharides) into oligosaccharides.

ANABOLIC STATE is a state where more body protein is being synthesized and deposited than is being broken down or destroyed. An untrained person is in anabolic neutral state. Training promotes a breakdown of muscle tissue which creates a demand for more protein. With more protein and calories in the diet along with rest, the body will compensate by laying down more protein creating an anabolic state. Too much training, insufficient rest, a lack of protein, or insufficient caloric intake will create a negative anabolic state.

ANABOLIC STEROIDS are derivatives of the male hormone testosterone or are derivatives of the female hormone progesterone. All steroids are a mix of "anabolic" and "androgenic" properties. Anabolic steroids tend to cause the body to store more protein in the muscle. This leads to larger and stronger muscles. With prolonged use, the body begins to adapt so the favorable protein balance lessens. At this point, the anabolic steroid continues to work by blocking cortisol absorption on the muscle. Cortisol is another stress hormone that causes the body to use more protein as a fuel source.

ANABOLISM is the build up of tissue either muscle

tissue or fat stores. Anabolism results when the body has sufficient protein, fatty acids, and energy to store these substances as fat or muscle. Training combined with a diet that provides a high amount of energy from carbohydrates and fat and sufficient amino acids from protein will favor muscle anabolism.

ANDROGEN typically means "male". Androgens refer to the male hormone testosterone. This hormone is responsible in men for their sex drive, aggression, height, large body size, and strength. Women also produce androgens/testosterone, but to a smaller degree. In the US, menopausal women are now being treated with minute amounts of testosterone to restore sex drive, and to increase energy levels. These are two of the biggest complaints of menopausal women.

ANDROGENIC HORMONES are the testosterone family. Testosterone is a powerful hormone produced by both males and females. Males produce 25 times the amount as females. This hormone is responsible for male sexual characteristics including facial hair, a deep voice, greater height, and aggression. While anabolic steroids have lesser androgenic/masculizing properties, the use will still increase secondary male characteristics. Athletes use these compounds along with anabolic steroids to increase protein retention in muscle. All steroids and hormones, when used in excess, will lower HDL levels, leading to cardiovascular risks.

ANDROSTENEDIONE is a steroid hormone naturally produced by the kidneys and is a precursor to testosterone. Some athletes use it to increase testosterone levels to aid muscle growth but it seems to be too weak to cause a significant change in testosterone levels.

ANTI-CATABOLIC Catabolism is the act of muscle wasting. Overtraining, eating too little calories, not eating enough protein, and doing too much aerobics when dieting all create a catabolic effect. This means the body is over stressed or under fed and tries to use its own muscle mass a fuel. In a catabolic situation, the body will tear down its own muscle to make more glucose. Anything that off sets catabolism is known to be an anti-catabolic agent. Common anti-catabolics, which prevent the body from using muscle as fuel, include branched chain amino acids, carbohydrate drinks, protein powders, OKG, and glutamine. The smart thing to do is to avoid overtraining, and to eat the right amounts of calories and protein to prevent a catabolic state in the first place.

ANTIDIURETIC HORMONE (ADH) is a hormone that is released by the kidneys in response to a low water intake. Many bodybuilders lower their water intake the final few days before a show in order to appear more cut. Lowering water intake too far will release ADH. ADH increases aldosterone levels which controls sodium and water levels in the body. The result of increasing ADH due to a low water intake is water retention!

ANTIOXIDANTS are substances that can fight and prevent the oxidation of organic molecules. A car left in a wet area will "oxidize" in time. It will rust and fall apart unless the owner treats the car with an anti-rust treatment. Well, exercise, smoke, pollution, stress, a high fat diet, and a high sugar diet all promote the production of unpaired electrons in the body. Left unchecked, these unpaired electrons can damage all tissues in the body and destroy anything they come in contact with, eventually leading to death. Fortunately, the body produces a few natural enzymes that combat these unpaired electrons/also known as free radicals. The back up fighters against free radicals include vitamins C, E and beta carotene. Supplementing with these nutrients can off set the detrimental effects of free radicals.

ANTI-VITAMIN This is a term used to describe anything that robs the body of vitamins or minerals. Alcohol can rob the body of vitamins, eating excessive protein can excrete calcium, drinking too much carbonated beverages can excrete phosphorous, and almost every prescription medicine causes the loss of at least one nutrient.

ARGININE is an individual amino acid that is "conditionally essential" meaning it is required during extreme high stress states or during growth periods. Babies require arginine to grow, as do hard training bodybuilders. Arginine gained its popularity as a growth hormone releaser as 30 grams of intravenous arginine in a hospital setting has been shown to increase growth hormone output and to accelerate wound healing. Thirty grams of oral arginine will give you diarrhea. The studies are mostly favorable showing 12 grams of arginine or 6 grams of ornithine taken on an empty stomach before sleep or hard training can increase GH levels. Some suggest adding choline to the arginine as it can inhibit the hormone somatostatin. Somatostatin is released to block excess GH release when GH releasers are used.

AROMATIZE is a term used to describe the process the body performs by making the female hormone estrogen from the male hormone testosterone. Males who use androgenic drugs like testosterone typically use an excessive amount. When the body is exposed to too much testosterone, the aromatase enzyme converts the testosterone to estrogen. It does so because the body wants a certain ratio of testosterone to estrogen (males produce both). When a bodybuilder injects a huge amount of testosterone, the body wants to raise its estrogen level to keep the ratio intact. It does this by converting some testosterone to estrogen. This process leads to severe water retention and the formation of gynecomastia, the feminizing of the breast tissue.

ASCORBIC ACID literally means "no scurvy" and is also known as vitamin C. Scurvy was a disease that was cured with the consumption or oranges over 200 years ago.

Ascorbic acid is a water soluble vitamin. While I suggest the bodybuilder get it every day from foods and supplemental form, the body does have the ability to store ascorbic acid. Vitamin C is necessary to help bind cells together, it strengthens blood vessel walls, it fights free radicals that destroy cells, it helps protect vitamins A and E in the body from invasive free radicals, and it strengthens the immune system and promotes healing and recovery. Women bodybuilders, who lose iron each month from their blood via menstruation need extra C as it increases the absorption of dietary iron. A high vitamin C intake is required to support the adrenal glands that often become severely overworked with hard training, and from using stimulants like Ma Huang.

Vitamin C is found in Citrus fruits and many vegetables and a bodybuilding favorite, potatoes. I suggest bodybuilders obtain 1 to 3 grams a day of vitamin C.

ASPARTIC ACID is one of the essential amino acids that is combined with glutamic acid to make aspartame, a sweetener used by those who wish to sweeten their food without the use of sugar. It yields 4 calories a serving compared to 16 calories of an equal amount of sugar.

ASPIRIN is a drug that is used in doses of 325 mg every other day as a maintenance precautionary to fight heart disease. Small amounts of aspirin block the production of chemical messengers called prostaglandins. One prostaglandin called PGE-2 produces thromboxane A2. Thromboxane A2 causes the blood to become too sticky. This leads to all sorts of heart ailments from heart attacks to strokes.

Aspirin also prolongs the effects of norepinephrine (NE). NE is released with the use of caffeine and ephedrine or Ma Huang to burn fat. Aspiring does this by blocking a prostaglandin that is released by the body to inhibit thermogenesis.

ATP is adenosine tri phosphate. ATP is the body's ultimate fuel source. The foods we eat are converted to ATP. ATP is used for digestion, muscle contraction, nerve transmission, and muscle growth. As the name implies, ATP is made of adenosine bonded to three phosphate molecules. When muscular work is employed, one of the molecules of phosphate is broken off to supply energy. This leaves us with ADP or adenosine di phosphate, or adenosine bonded with only two molecules of phosphate. To perform muscular work, the cells need ATP, not ADP. Therefore, the body makes more ATP from the remaining ADP plus creatine phosphate. This process of making more ATP takes 60 to 90 seconds in the body, so any bodybuilder should wait at least this amount of time before beginning a new set. The supplemental creatine that is popular can replenish creatine levels which in turn, when combined with ADP, make more ATP so the bodybuilder can perform more work.

—B—

BCAA include the amino acids leucine, isoleucine and valine. These amino acids are found in all animal source protein foods (chicken, meat, fish) but are found in highest concentrations in milk, milk products (yogurt and cheese) and eggs. They can be used as a back-up fuel source during weight training. The fuel source for weight training is primarily sugar from the blood and from muscle glycogen. When these two sources of fuel start to diminish, the body uses more protein (in the form of BCAA as fuel).

BEE POLLEN is a supplement that provides a wide array of many vitamins and minerals in a low dose.

BETA BLOCKERS are drugs that block the effects of the natural stress hormones in the body such as epinephrine. Athletes rely on drugs like ephedrine or clenbuterol for its stimulation. Ephedrine, clenbuetrol and other stimulants release stress hormones that increase fat breakdown and increase energy levels. Beta Blockers interfere with this reaction and effect.

BETA-CAROTENE is the vegetable source of vitamin A. It is found in yellow and orange colored vegetables. It is important in maintaining the protective linings of the stomach, intestines, and skin and it is required to make hormones in the body.

BETA SISTEROL is a plant sterol that is said to have anabolic properties in humans. No research has proven this to be true.

BETAINE HCL is a methyl donor also known as tri methyl glycine.

BIOFLAVINOIDS are antioxidants and are found in citrus fruits, usually with vitamin C. Bioflavanoids can fight bacteria, fight muscle inflammation and lower cholesterol. They also increase the absorption of vitamin C.

BIOTIN is a B-vitamin produced by the intestines or found in many foods. Egg yolks, liver, brown rice and beans are especially high in biotin. It is required to make growth hormone and testosterone. It is also required to use carbohydrates and fat as fuel. Theoretically, a low amount of biotin in the diet could impair fat metabolism.

BMR (basal metabolic rate) is the amount of calories a person needs in 24 hours doing ABSOLUTELY nothing. This is the energy needed to sustain muscle mass, and life in general. The body needs calories to keep the heart pumping, blood flowing and to perform the millions of chemical reactions required by the body. ANY additional movement requires calories. I call BMR "the total calories you need in a day staying in bed". To estimate BMR take your lean body mass in kg. (total bodyweight - fat weight = lean body mass) multiply by 2.2 and "add a zero". Example LBM = 100 kg x 2.2 = 220.
220 "+ zero" = 2200 calories

BLOOD SUGAR LEVELS is a description for the amount of sugar found in the blood stream. Normally the amount of sugar in the blood is 100 milligrams of glucose in 100 cubic centimeters of blood. This is commonly expressed as 100 milligrams percent. Blood sugar levels should not vary greatly above or below this number.

When meals are skipped or not enough carbohydrates consumed, the amount of sugar in the blood can fall. The body responds by releasing the hormone called glucagon which raises the amount of sugar in the blood. It does this by breaking down glycogen stores to obtain sugar. When too many carbs are eaten, and the amount of sugar in the blood increases, the body releases insulin which stores the excess glucose (sugar) as muscle glycogen or body fat.

BLOOD UREA NITROGEN is formed from the metabolism of proteins. Its rate of production in the body is correlated with protein breakdown. A very high protein diet or a bodybuilder who is losing muscle mass (in a catabolic state) due to strict dieting or overtraining will produce more blood urea.

BODY WEIGHT is a term used to describe the total mass (weight) one carries. It does nothing to tell a person how much fat or muscle he has.

BORAGE OIL is an oil that contains gamma linolenic acid (GLA). GLA is an intermediary (a by-product) of the natural breakdown of unsaturated fatty acids known as essential fatty acids. GLA can lead to many health benefits such as an increase in glutamine levels, improved growth hormone secretion, a positive nitrogen balance, and improved glucose tolerance. GLA can be obtained directly as a supplement from borage oil or it can be derived from unsaturated fatty acids. The body can not make GLA without essential fatty acids derived from the diet.

BORON is a trace mineral that is helpful in increasing bone density in women. Boron increases calcium absorption. Calcium supplements + boron + weight training is the best way to increase bone mass and to off set the disease called osteoporosis (bone thinning disease). Most diets supply about 1 to 2 milligrams a day of boron. 3-6 mg is the dose that may be helpful in building bone mass. It does NOT increase testosterone levels.

BREWER'S YEAST is a nutrient dense food that is high in chromium, zinc, and thiamine.

BROWN FAT is the special internal fat that supports the internal organs like the liver, heart, kidneys, and especially the lungs. Brown fat is not like white fat. White fat is the fat we all try to lose. White fat is found under the skin.

Brown fat is similar to muscles. Both are metabolically active. Both require calories for fuel. Training, stress, ephedrine and to a smaller degree, caffeine all stimulate brown fat.

BROWN RICE is a complex carbohydrate that is high in some B vitamins and relatively high in fiber.

BURNS is the name for short repetitions that cause the muscles to swell with blood. After failing with a weight, the bodybuilder would not be able to perform any more full reps, but he can shorten the range of motion on an exercise and perform smaller reps. When the muscles gorge with blood from burns, it sets in place a signal within the muscle that causes growth.

—C—

CAFFEINE is the drug found in coffee. It's cousin, theophylline is found in tea. Caffeine stimulates the nervous system. Bodybuilders use caffeine, especially when dieting. Drinking coffee before weight training can allow for a more forceful muscle contraction because the nervous system, which controls muscle contraction, becomes highly excited with caffeine consumption.

Coffee consumed before an aerobic workout will allow

the fat cell to break down easier. Caffeine stimulates hormone sensitive lipase, an enzyme that allows fat to leave the fat cell. This frees up more fatty acids to be used as fuel so the athlete can perform the aerobic exercise longer. In theory, using caffeine before aerobic exercise will allow more fat to be burned. The exception is when carbohydrates are eaten right before the aerobic session along with the caffeine. The sugar from the carbohydrates will off set the fat burning effects of the caffeine.

CALCIUM is a mineral required for strong bones and teeth. Ninety percent of the body's calcium is found in these two areas, the other one percent is found in the blood. The body needs more calcium during pregnancy, during childhood and during growth. Therefore bodybuilders need more calcium as calcium is needed in larger amounts in those who are growing.

Female bodybuilders should get plenty of calcium. As a female ages and produces less of the hormone, estrogen, the body's ability to absorb and use calcium becomes diminished.

Smoking, alcohol, and diet soda all decrease the body's ability to absorb calcium, while sunlight increases the absorption of calcium. Good sources are dairy products, and edible bones found in sardines and salmon. The best supplemental sources are calcium citrate and calcium carbonate.

Muscles need calcium in order to contract.

CALORIE is a unit of measure. It measures the amount of heat necessary to raise the temperature of a kilogram (one liter) of water one degree centigrade. The energy found in fat, carbohydrates, and protein is measured in calories. Calories may be used by the body to produce heat (thermogenesis) to build muscle, to enable the body to move, and to store body fat.

CALORIE DIET is weight loss diet based simply on eating less total calories. When a person eats less calories and therefore supplies less fuel to the body, the body will compensate by breaking down body fat so it can be used as fuel. All bodybuilding pre-contest diets are based on reducing calories. Some bodybuilders prefer to reduce carbohydrates to lower the calorie intake while others cut fat intake down to an absolute minimum in order to create a caloric deficit.

CANDIDA is a common bacterial infection that can be destroyed by using garlic capsules or by eating large amounts of garlic. Stress, antibiotics, birth control pills, pregnancy and diabetes can cause candida.

CARBOHYDRATES are a fuel source that regulate blood glucose levels. When carbohydrates are continually infused, the body will store the excess as muscle and liver glycogen. In an absence of carbohydrates, muscle and liver glycogen stores are disassembled to make glucose for the blood. Glucose is the main fuel source for weight training. The best choice is complex carbohydrates like pasta, rice, beans, and potatoes.

CARBOHYDRATE LOADING is a system used by bodybuilders the final week before a contest to allow for larger looking muscles. When carbohydrates are severely reduced and exhaustive exercise is employed, the muscle glycogen stores of carbohydrates become very very low. Carbohydrates attract water in the muscle. When carbohydrate stores are low, the muscles temporarily appear smaller than normal. But, this low level of carbs in the muscle sends the glycogen forming enzymes sky high.

When carbohydrates are reintroduced to the body or "loaded" nearly all of them will be stored quickly in the muscle. The bodybuilder can eat more carbohydrates than normal and not store them as fat. Any extra carbs will probably be stored in the muscle making them look bigger than before. Most bodybuilders restrict carbs for three days and exercise to failure. Then, they add back the carbohydrates into the diet the final three days before the contest.

CARBOHYDRATE THRESHOLD is the maximum amount of carbohydrates a bodybuilder can eat before storing body fat. Larger bodybuilders need more carbohydrates than smaller bodybuilders. When muscle glycogen levels are full, any extra carbohydrates consumed will be stored as fat as the muscles can no longer take any more carbs.

CARBON DIOXIDE is the end product of energy metabolism in the body from carbohydrates and fats. This by-product is excreted with the help of the lungs when we expel air.

CARNITINE is a nutrient that is NOT a fat burner. However, it does aid fat burning if you have stimulated fat breakdown in the first place with a calorie reduced diet or through exercise. Carnitine carries fatty acids into the mitocondria portion of muscle cells so that the fatty acids, already liberated from exercising or eating less, can be burned as fuel. Carnitine is not found in many foods. Lamb and organ meats are high in carnitine. Most bodybuilders use a supplemental dose of one to 3 grams daily while dieting.

CAROTENE is a precursor to vitamin A. Carotenoids are

yellow or orange in color and are found in foods that are yellow or orange such as squash, oranges, pumpkin, cantaloupe, sweet potatoes, carrots, and egg yolks. Carotenes are required for cell growth, skin and bone maintenance and to strengthen the membranes in the body. Vitamin A is also required by the body to produce growth hormone.

CATABOLIC STATE is a muscle losing state. The body begins to break down and use protein as fuel. It gets the protein from the amino acids found from foods in the diet and from lean muscle mass. Muscle can be broken apart by the body so the body can obtain fuel. Eating too few calories, not eating enough protein, or doing too much exercise with not enough rest all lead to a catabolic state.

CATABOLIC EXERCISE. Any exercise can be considered a catabolic exercise if the bodybuilder is in a catabolic state. If a bodybuilder is in a catabolic/muscle wasting state and trains with weights, the fuel required to perform the exercises comes from the body tearing apart its own muscle mass to supply fuel to do the exercises. The only way to get out of a catabolic state is to REST and do not do any exercise at all for at least three to five days. A feast way to lose muscle is to train when you are already in a muscle wasting state.

CATABOLISM is a muscle wasting or muscle destroying process that occurs in the body due to excess mental stress, excess physical stress, too few calories, or a lack of certain nutrients. Not eating enough protein, carbohydrates, avoiding essential fatty acids, or the lack of certain vitamins and minerals all can trigger a catabolic state. In a catabolic state hormones are released that destroy muscle tissue and organs to provide an alternative source of energy.

CELLULOSE is a fiber. It is the non digestible food substance found in the skins of fruits and vegetables.

CEREAL generally refers to oats, barley, wheat, corn, bulgar, and barley. These grains are high in B vitamins which are required to convert carbohydrates into usable fuel. These grains also are higher in fiber so they break down in the body at a slower pace than white flour.

CHITOSAN is a supplement that is made from the shells of shell fish like lobster, clams, mussels, and scallops. It can bind with fat in the blood and drag the fat out of the body so less is stored. Fiber works in the same say. While both chitosan and fiber do work - they bind with fat and pull it out of the blood leaving less fat remaining to be stored as body fat -, the amount of fat dragged out of the body is very small.

CHLORIDE is the negatively charged particle that is attached to sodium which is positively charged. Together, the positive of sodium attaches with the negative of chloride to form table salt NaC1, or sodium chloride. A deficiency in salt is very rare. Those inflicted with cystic fibrosis, an inherited disorder of the mucous producing glands in the pancreas, liver, and intestines, can lose large amounts of salt and must be careful not to become deficient.

CHOLERA is a bacteria that is common to cultures that have unsanitary living conditions. Cholera is found in microscopic amounts in feces and can live in warm water and food. It can be deadly, if it is not discovered and soon treated.

CHOLESTEROL is a waxy like substance related to fat. It helps the body to break down fats by making bile. The body can produce cholesterol. When cholesterol is lacking in the diet, the body manufactures more cholesterol. When a person eats a lot of cholesterol, the body reacts by making very little cholesterol. This self regulating system can fail with a high saturated fat diet, a high amount of body fat, or a diet that is low in fiber. When this occurs, cholesterol builds up and low density lipoproteins (LDL's) deposit the cholesterol on the sides of the cell walls leading to blockages and heart problems.

CHOLINE is a nutrient that is provided in the diet as a component of lecithin. Choline makes up acetylcholine, a neurotransmitter in the brain that makes a person feel more alert. Many bodybuilders use choline before training on an empty stomach to increase concentration. Choline also <u>inhibits</u> somatostatin, a messenger that <u>inhibits</u> grown hormone release. So, the bodybuilder using 1 to 2 grams of choline before training will feel more alert and release a little bit more growth hormone than normal.

CHONDROITIN is similar to glucosamine. It is derived from connective tissue and it adds flexibility to the joint tissue. 200 mg 3 times a day is suggested.

CHROMIUM is a trace mineral that is eliminated from the body in sweat due to a high sugar, high refined food diet that is low in fiber. Caffeine and steroids also eliminate chromium from the body.

Chromium can promote a mild increase in muscle and additional fat loss when used in conjunction with a good diet and training program. Chromium makes muscles more sensitive to insulin. Sensitive muscles use sugar better, making the body much better at storing carbohydrates as muscle glycogen. Sensitive muscle tissue also allows insulin to drive amino acids into the muscle tissue for growth and repair.

A sensitive muscle also means the body has to output LESS insulin. Lower insulin levels allow the body to tap fat as fuel while HIGH insulin levels (that occurs with non-insulin-sensitive muscle tissue) encourages the body to store carbohydrates as fat. Recommended dose: 200 mcg to 400 mcg daily.

CHROMIUM PICOLINATE is chromium that is attached to a niacin based molecule. This increases the absorption of chromium. Chromium Picolinate is the best source of chromium.

CITRIC ACID is another common name for vitamin C. Vitamin C is required in larger amounts by bodybuilders to fight the free radicals that are made from training hard, to support the immune system, and to aid in muscle recovery. Vitamin C can combat high amounts of cortisol, a stress hormone and catabolic hormone that is released with excessive training or with excessive dieting.

CLENBUTEROL is an asthma medication that stimulates beta receptors. Beta receptors are found on the lungs, so the asthmatic can breath easier as stimulating these beta receptors dilates the bronchi tubes leading to the lungs.

There are also beta receptors on fat and muscle. Clenbuterol can also stimulate these receptors. Stimulating the receptors on the muscle can decrease muscle breakdown that is associated with hard training and a calorie reduced diet. Stimulating the receptors on the fat cell will enable the fat cells to easily break down so that fat can be used as fuel and body fat stores can be reduced.

COBALT is part of the vitamin B-12 (cobalamin). Cobalt

is needed for red blood cell production and energy metabolism. It is found in spinach, cabbage, buckwheat, and lettuce.

CO-ENZYME are very small molecules that work with an enzyme to help that enzyme perform its job. Many enzymes in the body have B vitamins as part of their structure, so the B vitamins are also referred to as co-enzymes because they help enzymes do their job. A lack in B vitamins can inhibit the body from making enzymes. Here is how it looks: Co-enzyme + B vitamin + enzyme = An Enzyme (that can do its job)

CO-ENZYME Q-10 is a nutrient that has been shown to have heart protective properties by acting as an antioxidant, specifically targeting the heart tissue. Thirty mcg daily is the suggested dose.

COLLAGEN is a fibrous protein found in collagen fibers. Collagen fibers are the main support of connective tissue surrounding the joints, including tendons that hold muscles to the bones and ligaments that hold bones to bones.

Calcium, magnesium, vitamin C, and protein are 4 nutrients that provide nutritional support for these fibers.

COLOSTRUM is a thin yellow substance that is the precursor to breast milk. Colostrum can provide a breast feeding baby with several growth factors that promote the maturation and development of the baby. Among the factors in insulin-like growth factor, or IGF.

Colostrum is also found in small amounts in cow's milk leading some nutrition companies to make (bad) claims that this colostrum will work like human breast milk in supplying the body builder with IGF.

CONJUGATED LINOLEIC ACID (CLA) is a supplement that is gaining popularity. It is derived from saturated fats and has shown to act as a mild inhibitor of muscle inflammation. I think fish fat, or omega-3 fatty acids, work better and are dramatically less expensive. CLA has also been shown to prevent muscle breakdown by altering the prostaglandins in the body. This is a similar effect found with GLA and fish oils.

COPPER is a mineral that is required for proper formation of red blood cells and hemoglobin. Red blood cells transport oxygen between the lungs and body tissues (muscle) and carbon dioxide from the tissues to the lungs. The red blood cells contain hemoglobin which binds with iron and oxygen to assist in oxygen transport.

CORTISOL is a stress hormone that is released with stress, both too much physical or too much mental, and an extremely low calorie diet. Cortisol raises blood sugar levels by breaking down body protein. Body protein is converted to amino acids which are sent to the liver to be converted into glucose (blood sugar) to be used as fuel.

CREATINE MONOHYDRATE is a supplement that can increase creatine phosphate levels in the body. Increasing creatine phosphate levels allow more ATP to be made. All muscle contraction and muscle growth depends on adequate ATP levels. Insufficient levels of creatine phosphate leads to exhaustion and incomplete muscle recovery.

CREATINE PHOSPHATE is a high energy compound that acts as a reservoir or back up for the energy producing compound, ATP or adenosine triphophate.

All energy production, muscle building, and muscle contraction relies upon ATP. ATP is made from the foods we eat. Only a small amount of ATP is stored in the cells. Creatine phosphate is also stored in muscle. It is derived from foods especially red meat. When ATP is used as fuel, the body reduces the ATP to ADP. Creatine phosphate combines with ADP to make new ATP so more energy can be produced.

CREATININE is a by product produced when the kidneys are under a lot of stress. High creatinine levels can be found with blood tests administered by your doctor. A low water intake combined with a high protein diet could elevate these levels.

CYANOCOBALAMIN, also known as vitamin B-12, is found in meats and animal products only. Therefore, many vegetarians are severely deficient in this vitamin. The absorption of B-12 requires "intrinsic factor" - a compound made in the body. The intrinsic factor is located in the stomach. Here it attaches to the B-12 and carries it to the small intestine where it is released and fully utilized. At mid life, some unlucky people loose the intrinsic factor so absorption becomes impossible and B-12 must be injected into the body.

Low B-12 levels lead to anemia (low red blood cell count) and exhaustion. This is often mis-diagnosed as a deficiency in folacin.

CYCLOFENIL is a weak estrogen derived from plant sources. Cyclofenil will attach to estrogen receptors. This leaves stronger estrogens unable to attach to receptor cites (commonly found on fat cells) so body fat is less likely to be formed as estrogen is a known body fat storer. Lower estrogen levels also work to increase testosterone levels, so a male can lose some fat and add muscle due to a weaker estrogen being used by the body (remember the strong one is left inert because it can not bind to anything) and higher testosterone levels.

CYSTEINE is an amino acid that has immune stimulating properties. Cysteine is a precursor to glutathione. Whey protein is high in cysteine. Cysteine is found also in eggs and it is a component in hair.

CYSTINE refers to cystine stones which can form in the urinary tract and kidneys as the result of too much cysteine. Cysteine is water soluble but can oxidize into cystine which is insoluble in water. To prevent this make sure you supplement with vitamin C to prevent the oxidation of cysteine into cystine, especially if you eat a lot of eggs or use whey protein powders.

CYTOCHROME-C is an iron containing compound found in the mitocondria portion of a muscle cell. It is part of the electron transport system which derives ATP from foods.

—D—

DEFINITION is a term used to describe an incredibly low level of body fat attained by bodybuilders for competition.

DEHYDRATION results when the body lacks enough water to function. Bodybuilders who use steroids suffer from water retention that can blur muscle definition. Many use diuretics to lose water while others use diuretics and stop drinking fluids to lose water. This can be very dangerous. It will lead to severe muscle cramping. Bodybuilders who do not drink enough fluid can lower their metabolic rate, so fat loss becomes difficult.

DESSICATED LIVER is a supplement made of dried

liver. Since liver is probably the most nutrient dense foods on earth, dessicated liver is a great source of iron and B vitamins and several minerals.

DEXTRIN is a complex, long chain sugar, also known as maltodextrin which is a complex carbohydrate derived from corn. It breaks down and is absorbed slower than many carbohydrates and is the primary carbohydrate source in many meal replacement drinks like Met RX, NutriMet, and Rx Fuel.

DFA stands for **Dietary Fatty Acid**. There are essential fatty acids that we need to obtain from the diet because the body can not produce these fats. The fats are gamma linolenic acid and alpha linolenic acid and are required and involved in all the chemical reactions in the body.

DHA is found in cold water fatty fish like salmon, mackerel, and tuna. Omega-3's can improve cardiovascular function, reduce muscle inflammation, and improve the muscle tissue's ability to use glucose as fuel.

DHEA is a hormone produced from the adrenal glands in response to stress. It is also available in supplemental form. DHEA is broken down in the liver and produces adrogens (testosterone) in males and estrogen in females. Anecdotal reports indicate supplemental DHEA can increase energy levels and strength. DHEA levels begin to fall in both males and females after the age of 20.

DIBENCOZIDE is a form of vitamin B-12. B-12 is used by the body to produce energy. B-12 can be obtained in the diet, but absorption depends on "intrinsic factor" located in the digestive system. Unfortunately, many lack the ability to absorb B-12 due to impaired intrinsic factor.

This can lead to anemia. Dibencozide is a better absorbed form of B-12. It does not need the "intrinsic factor" to be absorbed. However, B-12 shots are the best way to obtain B-12.

D

DIET is the term used to describe all the foods a person eats on a daily basis. The low fat diet is the most popular diet where a person eats foods that are lower in fat. A low sugar diet is the diet preferred by diabetics while bodybuilders eat a diet that is high in complex carbohydrates and protein and low in fat.

DIETARY FIBER is a non digestible food substance found in plants. Humans lack the enzymes to break down fiber. However, fiber is definitely important. It adds "bulk" to the diet and improves the vitality of the intestines. It can also decrease food intake and caloric intake for dieters as it adds no calories to the diet. Fiber also can lower blood sugar levels by slowing the release of sugars form carbohydrate foods from the gut into the blood.

DIMETHYL SULFOXIDE (DMSO) is a solvent used in making paper. It is a very strong anti oxidant that has been used to fight muscle inflammation, and improve joint pain. It is transdermal when rolled onto the skin. This means it can penetrate and go right through the skin.

DIMETHGLYCINE (DMG) is a methyl donor. Methyl groups in the body (found naturally in metabolism) increase the efficiency of muscle metabolism. People who use DMG think they can increase muscle performance by adding DMG, but the body doesn't increase methyl groups by supplementing. Only exercise can add/increase more methyl donors to the body.

DIOSTEROL is a synthetic hormone that mimics the female hormone estrogen.

DIPEPTIDE is a term used to describe the way amino acids are joined together in whole protein foods. When a bodybuilder eats eggs, chicken, or fish (whole protein foods) the amino acids are broken off two pieces (or two amino acids) at a time. These two aminos, called dipeptide, are then absorbed by the small intestine. Dipeptide absorption is the way the body best uses amino acids. For muscle growth, single free form amino acids are inferior as they are single in nature, and the way the body is set up for amino acids utilization is two aminos (dipeptide) at a time.

DNA a long molecule found in every cell in the body. It is the master code that is used by the body to produce every other molecule in the body. It is commonly referred to as a person's genetic code or "genetic blueprint" as everyone has a slightly unique DNA.

DOPING is the word to describe an athlete who has used drugs to enhance his performance. Steroids, amphetamines, and the drug EPO can be considered doping. (EPO increases blood volume - so an athlete can deliver more oxygen to the tissues for aided performance and faster recovery.)

DOPING CHECK is drug testing to screen for the above drugs. The popular doping tests are urine analysis and blood analysis.

—E—

ECTOMORPH is one of the three body types. Ectomorph have very slight or small muscles in an untrained state, very little body fat, and a small bone structure. Ectomorphs can build muscle, but genetically, it is almost impossible to build huge amounts of muscle. There are no pure ectomorphs competing today on the professional mens level. Flex Wheeler has a small ectomorph bone structure, but his muscles are mesomorphic in nature; they are round, full and long in shape.

EICOSAPENTAENOIC ACID (EPA) is a substance found in fish oils. These oils are called omega-3 fatty acids. Omega-3 fatty acids exert a hormonal effect on the body. They produce prostaglandins, hormone like messengers, that make the muscle cell more sensitive to the effects of the hormone insulin. Recall, insulin is a hormone that drives amino acids and sugar found in the blood into muscles cells to aid in recovery and growth. Omega-3 fatty acids work similar to the trace mineral chromium. The muscle becomes very sensitive to the insulin. This means the body can effectively drive aminos and carbohydrates into muscle cells. Also, a sensitive muscle cell to insulin means that less total insulin has to be released. High insulin levels are correlated with obesity. Omega 3 fatty acids also produce polyamines in the body. Polyamines are important regulators of cell growth and have been shown to promote protein synthesis. Lastly, fish oils can preserve muscle glutamine levels.

ELECTROLYTES are salts that allow for electrical transfer of currents in the body. The three electrolytes are potassium, chloride, and sodium. Potassium is found inside cells while sodium and chloride are found outside of cells.

EMPTY CALORIE is calories that provide little or no

nutrition at all. There are many different types of empty calories. Alcohol is definitely a source of empty calories. First it provides calories with no nutrition at all. Second, it robs the body of several vitamins and minerals by causing the excretion of these nutrients. Sugar can be considered an empty calorie food as it provides calories and carbs, with no other significant source of vitamins and minerals. Many "junk foods" are also considered a source of empty calories. For example, one donut, or one candy bar, may provide 180 to 225 calories, plenty of sugar and fat, no complete protein and no significant source of any one vitamin or mineral. The problem with empty calorie foods is that studies show they displace other foods. That is, people do not eat healthy foods and eat donuts or drink alcohol on top of the healthy foods. Instead, they eat donuts, candy, cookies, sweets, and other empty calorie foods without eating any healthy foods that supply plenty of vitamins, minerals, and nutrition that the body requires.

ENDOMORPHY is a term to describe a genetic body type. Endomorphs have large bone mass, a large amount of muscle mass, and a larger amount of fat mass. The two other genetic body types are ectomorph and mesomorph.

ENERGY is derived from the three macronutrients, carbohydrates, fat, and protein. One gram of carbohydrates yields 4 calories of energy, one gram of fat yields 9 calories and one gram of protein yields 4 calories. Bodybuilders use a large amount of carbohydrates during workouts as the fast twitch type 2 b muscle fibers prefer sugar as a fuel. Some of this energy comes from glucose in the blood. When blood glucose levels fall, the body begins to use glucose that is stored in the muscles called muscle glycogen. If muscle glycogen levels are low, the workouts become less intense as the type 2b fast twitch fibers lack the correct fuel source. Fats are the main source of energy used during aerobic exercise. Protein can be used as fuel, to a smaller degree during both weight training and aerobic training. Not consuming enough fuel will inhibit the bodybuilder's ability to train hard and grown.

ENERGY SOURCE refers back to carbohydrates, protein, and fat. These are the three sources of fuel for the human body. ATP, the body's ultimate source of fuel on the cellular level is derived from foods.

EPHEDRA and EPHEDRINE are sympatomimetics which means they stimulate the sympathetic nervous system. Stimulating the sympathetic nervous system can have three beneficial effects to the bodybuilder. First, the appetite becomes mildly suppressed. Second, nerves fire with more force, thereby making muscle contractions more forceful and powerful. Third, the nervous system indirectly governs fat metabolism. Any time the sympathetic nervous system is stimulated the metabolic rate speeds up making it easier to burn more calories. Using ephedrine could increase the metabolic rate by 5% to 7%, decrease appetite by 10% to 15%, and promote more forceful muscle contractions during training sessions.

EPINEPHRINE is a one of the two catecholamine hormones released from the adrenal medulla situated atop the kidneys. Epinephrine stimulates the nervous system increasing blood pressure and heart rate. It also causes the muscle to break apart the sugar that is stored in the muscles as muscle glycogen, so it can be used as a fuel. It also allows fat cells to release fatty acids so fat loss becomes somewhat easier. Epinephrine also can suppress the appetite. Epinephrine is released in stressful situations and during hard weight training workouts.

ESSENTIAL AMINO ACIDS are the 8 amino acids the body can not make. The essential 8 amino acids must be consumed each day from protein foods. The body requires the 8 essential amino acids to make hormones, enzymes, antibodies, and support the immune system. Muscular growth is impossible without these 8 amino acids.

ESSENTIAL FATTY ACIDS (EFA's) are derived from vegetable oils. They can not be made by the body and must be consumed in the diet for normal growth. Bodybuilders who follow a completely zero fat diet will develop essential fatty acid deficiencies which will prevent muscle growth. EFA's are precursor to hormone like substances called eicosnoids which are essential for growth.

ESTROGEN is the hormone that is predominantly produced by females, in the ovaries, though males also produce estrogen, to a much smaller degree. The role of estrogen in females is to stimulate growth and development. Estrogen is responsible for the females breasts and reproductive system. Estrogen is also one reason why women carry more body fat, particularly in the lower body and hips. Males who abuse steroids often develop enlarged breasts due to an excess intake of testosterone. The body tries to regulate itself by converting some testosterone into estrogen. Finally, estrogen can cause severe water retention in many individuals.

EVENING PRIMROSE OIL contains gamma linoleic

acid (an omega-6 fatty acid) a precursor to "healthy" prostaglandins that can fight muscle inflammation, increase growth hormone output and increase blood flow to muscles.

—F—

FAST GLYCOLYTIC FIBER are considered the fast twitch type 2b fibers. They fatigue very easily, but can generate the largest amount of force. These fibers are best suited for rapid and explosive quick movements that generate power. They use exclusively glucose as fuel. These fibers come into play with the use of heavy weights lifted to failure in the 4 to 12 rep range. They have the greatest potential for muscle hypertrophy.

FAST OXIDATIVE GLYCOLYTIC FIBER are considered the fast twitch type 2a fibers. During exercise these fibers can use a mix of fat or glucose as fuel. If there is little stored muscle glycogen in the body, the fibers will try to use more fat for fuel. These fibers are moderately resistant to fatigue and can generate dramatically more power than slow twitch fibers but less power than the fast glycolytic fibers. These are the types of muscle fibers used in sets that are of higher reps, 15 or more.

FAST TWITCH FIBER are muscle fibers that use predominantly sugar or glucose as fuel, though they are capable of using fat as well. Fast twitch muscle fibers have the greatest capacity for muscle hypertrophy (growth). There are two types of fast twitch fibers. Type 2a and type 2b. The 2b fibers respond best to bodybuilding training, 4 to 12 reps to failure, and use sugar exclusively for fuel. These fibers fatigue easily in response to heavy weights. They can grow by as much as 100%, so a 12 inch arm can theoretically grow into a 24 inch arm.

FAT is a term used to describe either lipids or body fat. Dietary fat is found in oil, butter, all protein foods and to a lesser degree in complex carbohydrates. Dietary fat provides nine calories per gram of fat.

Body fat is generally the result of eating too many carbohydrates and too much dietary fat. Body fat and dietary fats look similar in that they are classified as triglycerides. A triglyceride is one molecule of glycerol attached to three fatty acids.

FAT LOADING is a technique used the final 3 days before a bodybuilding contest to aid in carbing up the muscles. Fats slow digestion and also slow the breakdown of carbohydrates. When a bodybuilder carbs up for a contest, his goal is to make the muscles appear bigger and tighter. Most bodybuilders use complex carbohydrates as a carbohydrate source during the loading period since they break down slower and cause less water retention. Adding fat to the diet slows carb break down and prevents water retention. Fats also restore intra-muscular fat (the fat inside muscles - not the fat under the skin) which can also add to muscle fullness. Dieting decreases both fat stores under the skin and fat stores in the muscle.

FAT SOLUBLE VITAMINS are members of the lipid family. They are vitamins A, D, E, and K and all are absorbed with dietary fat. They travel around in the body with the help of fats, and they can be stored by the body. Any disease that produces fat malabsorption can bring about a deficiency in the fat soluble vitamins.

FATTY ACID is an organic acid composed of a carbon chain with hydrogen atoms attached. It is a part of dietary fat and body fat.

FATTY LIVER describes the early stage of liver deterioration. Liver deterioration occurs when the liver is taxed and abused from eating too many fatty foods, or from drinking an excessive amount of alcohol for a long period of time, or from taking steroids for an extended period of time. Fatty liver is characterized by accumulation of fat in liver cells.

FEEDBACK describes the body's built in system of "checks and balances". For example, when you drink too little water, the body reacts by holding water. When you drink an excessive amount of water, the body excretes water.

FILAMENTS are the microscopic actin and myosin filaments that comprise each individual muscle fiber. The actin and myosin filaments are proteins and are responsible for muscle contraction, and thicken in size due to weight training.

FISH OILS contain omega-3 fatty acids which make the receptor for insulin on the muscle more sensitive so less insulin is released in response to eating carbohydrates. Moderate insulin levels inhibit fat storage and encourage an anabolic environment by driving carbohydrates and amino acids from protein foods into muscle cells. Fish oils also buffer muscle inflammation and can spare muscle glutamine levels.

5-HTP is also known as 5-hydroxy-L-trytophan. It is a naturally occurring metabolite derived from the amino acid tryptophan. It has been shown to promote sleep and increase Growth Hormone output.

FLUORINE is a trace mineral that is found in drinking water or added to drinking water that is naturally very low in fluorine. With the help of calcium, vitamin D, zinc, manganese and boron, it is required to make strong bones and teeth.

FREE FORM AMINO ACID are amino acids that are "free" of any other amino acid. Normally, in foods, amino acids are bonded together two at a time. After the small intestines absorb amino acids that are linked together in pairs, the pairs are broken into individual "free" amino acids. Supplement companies sometimes manufacture free form amino acids in hopes they are superior in absorption and muscle growth.

FREE RADICALS are unstable oxygen atoms or molecules that are produced with exercise and can damage everything they touch. They can promote diabetes and damage the immune system. Vitamins A, C and E, selenium, zinc, glutathione, Coenzyme Q10 all fight the negative effects of free radicals.

FRUCTOSE is the main type of sugar found in fruits. When it is bound with glucose, it forms sucrose, the sugar found in sugar cane. Fructose is sometimes used by bodybuilders as a sweetener in baking or as a sweetener in oats because it does not, calorie for calorie, illicit as much insulin release than other sugar like cane sugar.

—G—

GALACTOSE is a simple sugar. Simple sugars are known as monosaccharides. Mono means one and saccharide means sugar. The other mono saccharides are fructose found in fruits and glucose. Galactose and glucose combine to make lactose, the sugar found in milk.

GAMMA ORYZANOL is a derivative of rice bran oil. It

is thought to increase testosterone levels in the body. However, there also is evidence that it may <u>decrease</u> testosterone levels.

GAMMA LINOLEIC ACID (GLA) is a special type of fat found in borage oil. GLA also can aid in fat loss by making brown fat (the fat surrounding the internal organs - the fat that is metabolically active) more sensitive to adrenalin. This promotes an increase in thermogenesis.

GARCINIA CAMBOGIA is derived from tamarind, a fruit found in Africa and many Middle Eastern countries. When carbohydrates are over eaten, the body releases too much insulin which in turn sends a message to certain enzymes to make body fat from the excess carbohydrate intake. Garcinia temporarily interrupts the enzyme ATP citric lyase. Citric lyase can form acetyl coenzyme A which will take the extra carbs and store them as body fat.

Another benefit of garcinia is that it shunts the excess carbs somewhere else; mainly toward both the liver and muscle so glycogen stores can stay high. High glycogen stores are helpful in recovery. Most bodybuilders use 250 mg of hydroxycitric acid 3 to 4 times a day, twenty minutes before a high carb meal. Some build up to a 1000 mg dose.

GERM OIL comes from wheat. It contains the polyunsaturated fatty acid called linoleic acid which promotes the release of "local hormone like substances" called eicosanoids. Eicosanoids can improve immunity and fight muscle inflammation.

GERM RICE is the very outer most portion of brown rice providing fiber, minerals, vitamins, and an incomplete but high source of protein.

GINKO BILOBA is an herb that can increase blood flow to the brain and it has been shown to improve short term memory.

GINSENG is an "adaptogen". Adaptogens allow the body to recover faster and better from stress, both physical and mental stress. Ginseng may increase stamina and recovery as many athletes have reported feeling better after using ginseng. Several studies support these claims as ginseng has been shown to improve oxygen consumption by working muscles and stimulate receptors in the brain promoting a strong mental sense of arousal.

GLANDULARS are supplements derived from grinding up organs of animals, usually cows or bulls. It is believed that taking the thyroid of a cow can somehow increase the thyroid levels in the blood of a bodybuilder. Others use glandulars of adrenal glands to obtain more energy or take glandulars derived from bulls testicles to obtain more testosterone. I doubt there can be any beneficial effect from using these types of supplements.

GLOBULIN is a type of protein found in the blood that helps to transport calcium, fats, iron, drugs, or act as buffers in the blood to keep the ph in the blood at 7.4.

GLUCONEOGENESIS means "the production of new sugar". Normally, the hard working muscles of a bodybuilder rely on glucose as fuel. If there is a lack of glucose in the blood and muscle glycogen stores are low, the body will make glucose from proteins. Some of these proteins are found in the blood as amino acids from an earlier meal. Or, the body can tap muscle, which is made of protein, and break it apart to obtain sugar to be used as fuel.

GLUCOSAMINE helps to stimulate the production of cartilage, (the joint tissue is made of tendons and ligaments). It also has an anti-inflammatory effect on the connective tissue - so it may be helpful to bodybuilders 500 - 1000 mg of glucosamine taken 3 times a day seems to work best.

GLUCOSAMINE SULFATE is involved in the formation of joint tissue. Bodybuilders can benefit from using it as it strengthens and lubricates the joints.

GLUCOSE is a monosaccharide that is often referred to as "blood sugar". It is the sugar that all cells use for fuel. Any carbohydrate food contains glucose and grape juice is pure glucose. Bodybuilders should eat smaller meals that are moderate in carbohydrate intake to maintain normal blood sugar levels. Too many carbs will flood the blood with too much glucose and much of the glucose will be stored as fat. Skipping meals will lower blood glucose levels which in turn triggers the body to use protein as a fuel source.

GLUTAMIC ACID is a precursor to glutamine in the body. Glutamine is required to support immunity and to provide a back up in fuel during catabolic states. Low muscle glutamine levels are associated with a lack of muscle growth. The best source of glutamine is from the protein foods. Supplementary glutamic acid is not a good idea as little glutamic acid by itself is not converted to glutamine in the body. Glutamic acid derived from whole foods can be converted to glutamine.

GLUTAMINE is an amino acid that makes up 50 to 60% of the total amino acids found in muscles. It is used to off set the negative effects of ammonia that is produced with hard workouts. When the body is stressed, glutamine leaves the muscles and is sent into the blood to support the immune system. It is the "immunity amino acid" - it supports the immune system. Immune support is more important than muscle growth for survival. The immune system must be supported first before muscle growth can occur. Low muscle glutamine levels means no muscle growth. Glutamine, like all amino acids, produce ammonia BUT it decreases more ammonia than it produces. The net effect is LESS ammonia.

GLUTATHIONE is an antioxidant that has effects throughout the body. It has especially strong free radical fighting effects in the liver. Some research shows that glutathione can inhibit a fatty liver from developing. Glutathione levels can be raised by using whey protein or using an individual supplement. Look for one that provides 100 mg in a daily dose.

GLYCEMIC INDEX describe the rate at which carbohydrate foods increase blood sugar levels and insulin in the body. Some carbohydrate foods break down in the body faster than others. When this occurs, the body responds by outputting too much insulin. High blood insulin levels tend to strongly influence fat storage. Lower blood sugar levels promote a smaller output of insulin. Lower insulin levels have an anabolic effect without causing fat storage. Bodybuilders should eat 5 to 6 smaller meals which forces the bodybuilder to eat only a moderate amount of carbohydrates and food at any one sitting. This controls insulin levels. Also fiber and the small amounts of fat found in protein foods tends to slow the breakdown of carbohydrate foods into the blood leaving a smaller output in insulin than if carbohydrates where consumed alone.

Stay away from desserts, processed foods, white flour, fruit juices, rice cakes, and even white rice. All break down fast in the body.

GLYCEROL is a molecule that combines with 3 fatty acids to make fat. When a bodybuilder refers to body fat or when we refer to dietary fat we are talking about triglycerides . . . 3 fatty acids (tri) combined with glycerol. Supplementqal glycerol is used to hydrate the body and excrete sodium from the body.

GLYCINE is a single amino acid that has been shown to increase growth hormone when given in 3 to 6 gram dosages on an empty stomach before weight training workouts.

GLYCOGEN is a form of stored carbohydrates. When an excess amount of carbohydrates are eaten, the body can store them as fat or glycogen. Glycogen stores are found in both the liver and muscles. High glycogen stores are correlated with faster muscle recovery. When glycogen stores are high and the bodybuilder has missed a meal and is in the gym training hard, the muscles can release some of this stored glycogen into the blood as glucose. If muscle glycogen stores are low and the bodybuilder did not eat enough carbohydrates and starts to train, the body will use protein as a fuel source. Some of this protein comes from muscle as muscle is made of protein.

GLYCOLYSIS is a process by which glucose is converted to pyruvic acid. Weight training is an anaerobic exercise. Anaerobic means oxygen is not present. When you are training with weights glucose is converted to pyruvic acid which in turn is converted into lactic acid. Lactic acid can be converted back to pyruvic acid and eventually used as fuel.

With aerobic exercise, glucose is converted to pyruvic acid which then enters the krebs cycle to yield energy.

GROWTH HORMONE is released in the brain when the body is exposed to deep sleep, low blood sugar levels, stress, or the amino acid arginine. Growth hormone increases protein synthesis and it causes the fat cells to more readily break down so the body can obtain additional fuel. Growth hormone also increases insulin like growth factors (IGF) in the liver which also promotes protein synthesis.

—H—

HARD GAINER is a term used to describe a person who has a very difficult time adding lean body mass. A hard gainer is usually an ectomorph - a person who is genetically slightly muscled, with very little body fat and a fast metabolism.

HCG (HUMAN CHORIONIC GONADOTROPIN) is a protein hormone derived from the placenta of a pregnant woman. It is used by male bodybuilders to increase testosterone levels.

When a male uses synthetic testosterone or anabolic steroids, the body shuts down a hormone in the brain called luteinizing hormone. This hormone is responsible for signaling the testes to produce testosterone. The testes stop making testosterone because there is an additional or alternative source, the steroids being injected. After stopping steroids, the male body usually will not immediately begin to produce luteinizing hormone so testosterone can not be produced. Therefore, the bodybuilder often chooses to use HCG which will increase his own testosterone level by stimulating the release of luteinizing hormone.

HDL CHOLESTEROL is a protein carrier in the blood. Cholesterol is a fatty like substance and the blood through which it travels is a watery substance. In order for the cholesterol to travel through the blood, it must attach itself to a protein carrier. Of the four carriers, HDL or high density lipoproteins are the most "helpful". HDL cholesterol carries cholesterol to the liver where it can be destroyed. The "bad" cholesterol, LDL's deposits cholesterol on the artery walls, leading to heart disease. Exercise, a diet that contains fish oils, garlic, onions, a high fiber intake, a stress free lifestyle, and having plenty of muscle mass, all increase HDL levels.

HIGH DENSITY LIPOPROTEIN (HDL) is a protein carrying molecule in the body that carries cholesterol from the blood back to the liver where this excessive cholesterol can be destroyed. Low HDL levels lead to blocked arteries and heart attacks. Training, a high fiber diet, chromium, fish oils, a low fat and low saturated fat diet, and garlic all favor a high productions of HDLs.

HIGH FAT DIET is a diet used to shed fat. It requires the dieter to do two things: cut way back on carbohydrates and at the same time increase dietary fat. However for the diet to be successful, the dieter must eat less total calories than he was previously eating in order to lose fat.

Lowering carbs will lower insulin levels. Low insulin levels allows for fat breakdown. Dietary fat breaks down slower than carbohydrates so it makes the dieter feel "full" after eating.

HIGH PROTEIN DIETS are used to build muscle and to lose fat. All bodybuilders who want to gain muscle must eat enough protein to add muscle mass. I recommend 1 gram of protein per pound of lean muscle mass. This amount is high for the normal/non active person. Protein is needed in higher amounts to build muscle. The more muscle you carry, the more protein you need.

A high protein diet is also needed during dieting as excess protein can be used as fuel. If the bodybuilder is dieting and does not eat enough protein, the body will call upon muscle. The body will break down muscle mass to obtain the branched chain amino acids which are needed by the dieting bodybuilder as a backup fuel source.

HISTADINE is an essential amino acid important for growth in babies, and pre-pubescent children. As adults, we are capable of making histadine from the 8 essential amino acids. Some supplement companies add histadine to its protein powders along with arginine as both are required when the body is growing (ie childhood and pregnant mothers) and bodybuilders are similar in that they are adding stress to the body and the body is also growing.

HMB is a derivative of leucine, the most important branched chain amino acid. Leucine can prevent muscle breakdown and be used as fuel by working muscles that are low in muscle glycogen. HMB has been shown to work similar to leucine. Bodybuilders who run the risk of losing muscle, such as those dieting for competition, could benefit from HMB. Beware, the cost is high.

HORMONES are part of the body's Endocrine System. There are three categories: 1) hormones made of amino acids like epinephrine or melatonin 2) hormones made from (poly) peptides like insulin and 3) hormones made from steroids like testosterone or estrogen. Hormones are secreted in one part of the body and flow through the blood to target other areas of the body. For example, the brain releases Luteinizing hormone which travels through the blood and targets the testes (in males) to make testosterone.

HYDROCHLORIC ACID is secreted into the stomach to break down protein foods into smaller chains of amino acids for absorption.

HYDROXYCITRATE is found either in supplemental form or in fruits like tamarind native to South America, Africa, and the Middle East. Hydroxycitrate is a fat inhibitor. It works by inhibiting the enzyme ATP citrate lyase which can store fat from carbohydrates.

HYPOGLYCEMIA is also known as low blood sugar. Avoiding carbohydrates, eating less calories, and exercise all lower the amount of sugar in the blood. When low blood sugar occurs the body releases a hormone called glucagon. Glucagon increases the amount of sugar in the blood by breaking down stored muscle and liver glycogen. Liver and muscle glycogen is split and sent into the blood as glucose to combat the low sugar level.

—I—

IMMUNITY SYSTEM is the body's complex defense system that is activated to fight off bacteria, virus and other foreign substances that may be harmful to the body. A low fat diet, exercise and a good diet that provides adequate glutamine, vitamins C, E, beta carotene, riboflavin, folacin, zinc, and selenium support a strong immune system. Bodybuilders who use steroids or over train and over diet often weaken the immune system and lose muscle and more easily catch colds and feel exhausted.

INOSINE is a purine nucleotide that promotes oxygen transport. This could give a user more energy. It is also used to increase ATP levels similar, but inferior to that of creatine.

INOSITOL can be made by the body, supplied by the diet, and is popular in supplemental form. It contributes to lipid or fat metabolism by preventing a fatty liver. It allows the liver to manage the metabolism of fats. Food sources include grapefruits, melons, oranges, beans, and green beans.

INSULIN is a protein hormone secreted by the pancreas. When carbohydrates are consumed they are digested and sent to the blood stream. All carbohydrates eventually are broken down into glucose. The job of insulin is to remove the glucose from the blood. Insulin drives glucose into the muscles to form muscle glycogen. However, if muscle glycogen stores are full, or if a large or excess amount of glucose is present in the blood, insulin will divert the glucose towards fat cells. Insulin also is responsible for channeling amino acids from the blood into the muscle. Being a carbohydrate and amino acid storer, insulin has become known as an "anabolic hormone".

INVERTED SUGAR is the name of a solution that is 50% glucose and 50% fructose. It is obtained from the breakdown of sucrose. Sucrose is called "table sugar" or cane sugar. It is the one found in restaurants to sweeten coffee and tea.

IRON is a mineral that is found in both vegetables and meat, but the (red) meat source is dramatically better because it is easiest to absorb. Iron is needed for energy production and for the formation of red blood cells.

IRON DEFICIENCY ANEMIA results when the body lacks iron. When the body lacks iron, red blood cells contain less hemoglobin. Hemoglobin carries blood, nutrients, and oxygen to tissues. Low iron leads to exhaustion and a decreased metabolic rate.

ISOLEUCINE is one of the three branched chain amino acids. The other two are valine, and leucine. The branched chain amino acids can be used directly by the muscle as fuel during training sessions, when carbohydrates are lowered (like before a contest) or during prolonged aerobic work. The BCAA are also known as anti-catabolics. Using them before training will allow the muscle to use the supplemental form of BCAA. If there are no BCAA in the blood, working muscle may break itself apart to obtain BCAA because muscles are made of BCAA! Use a supplement to create an anti-catabolic environment.

—J—

JUNK FOOD is referred to any man made food that provides lots of fat or sugar without any other nutritional value. Snack foods like candy bars, cakes, and most desserts are classified as junk food.

—K—

KAVA KAVA is a plant native to the South Pacific. It is a mild diuretic and muscle relaxant. Users report a feeling of "well-ness" and also dream "clearer" when they sleep.

KELP is a mineral that is required to support a normal thyroid function.

KETOISOCARPOATE (KIC) is a keto acid (a cousin) to the branched chain amino acid Leucine. When muscle glycogen stores are low, the body requires more branched chain aminos as a fuel. KIC also works like the branched chain amino acids but it is better. KIC acts as an ammonia scavenger. Ammonia is produced with muscle breakdown or with a high protein diet. Ammonia interferes with ATP production, muscle contraction, and glycogen formation. Using KIC, especially when dieting for a show can prevent muscle breakdown while lowering ammonia levels.

—L—

LACTATE MECHANISM describes the body's use of lactate during exercise. In the lactic acid system (also known as anaerobic metabolism) pyruvic acid is produced when glucose is used by the working muscles. Pyruvic acid is converted into lactic acid which accumulates and builds up in the muscle because the muscles can not directly use lactate. When a person stops exercising, the lactic acid in the muscles are sent to the liver where it is converted back to pyruvate which can be made back into sugar (glucose).

LACTIC ACID is a byproduct of carbohydrate breakdown. The working and contracting muscles of a bodybuilder use glucose from the blood or from muscle glycogen as fuel to make ATP - the real fuel of muscle. When ATP is formed from glucose, lactic acid is also formed. Lactic acid can cause fatigue and prevent fat breakdown. Between sets, lactic acid is sent to the liver and eventually converted to glucose.

LACTIC ACID SYSTEM is also known as anaerobic metabolism. Anaerobic means "without oxygen" and is the metabolic system used in weight training. The fuel in the lactic acid/anaerobic system is glucose, pyruvate and lactate. Pyruvate and lactate are byproducts of glucose metabolism. When an exercise continues for more than two minutes, the lactic acid system gives way to the aerobic system where fat is the primary fuel source.

LACTIC ACID THRESHOLD is the maximum lactic acid the muscles can handle before the lactic acid produced from high intensity exercise interferes with muscle contraction. Regular weight training can increase a muscle's lactic acid threshold.

LACTOSE is the form of sugar found in milk and milk products. It is broken down into glucose to create "blood sugar". As adults age, they loose the ability to break down and metabolize lactose. This is sometimes referred to as "lactose intolerance".

LDL CHOLESTEROL Cholesterol is a fatty like substance produced by the body. Cholesterol is required to build bile salts which are released from the gallbladder to break down dietary fat and to build sex hormones. Cholesterol is not found in plants. It is found in animal flesh like beef, lamb, fish, and milk. The body can make its own cholesterol if dietary cholesterol intake is restricted. When a healthy person eats too much cholesterol, the body reacts by producing less cholesterol. In a healthy person who avoids cholesterol, the body reacts by manufacturing more. Controllable factors that can interfere and destroy this natural self regulating mechanism is smoking, drugs, anabolic steroids, a high saturated fat diet, a lack of exercise, and being overweight.

There are two types of cholesterol in the body. "Good" cholesterol is referred to as HDL or high density lipoprotein. "Bad" cholesterol is referred to a LDL or low density lipoprotein. Since cholesterol is a fat like substance, it must be carried through the watery bloodstream by a carrier. HDLs carry cholesterol from the blood to the liver where they are destroyed. HDLs can also shunt cholesterol towards bile where the body excretes it. LDLs carry cholesterol from the blood and deposits it on the walls of the cells. Most of these cells line arteries that carry blood from the heart. Once the cholesterol is deposited on the walls, scarring occurs, and the walls begin to narrow impeding blood flow, leading to various cardiovascular problems.

A favorable HDL to LDL ratio is the goal. Many people can have low amounts of cholesterol in the body, but are at risk for cardiovascular disease since the HDL are low and LDL are too high. It is also possible to have very high amounts of cholesterol in the body and be in perfect health as long as LDLs are in check and HDLs are high.

Common antioxidants, especially vitamin E can inhibit the scarring that takes place when LDLs deposit cholesterol on cell walls.

LECITHIN is found in every cell in the body. It helps break down cholesterol and contain the lipotropics known as choline and inositol. Lecithin helps the body break down fat. It is a part of bile. Bile is made by the liver. When you eat fat, the body releases bile to break down and absorb the dietary fat.

LEUCINE is the most important branched chain amino acid. It can be used by working muscle as fuel to make ATP and it increases the release of insulin which prevents muscle breakdown and increases muscle (protein) synthesis.

LINOLENIC ACID is derived from the essential fatty

acid called linoleic acid. Linoleic acid is found in vegetable oils. Linolenic acid is found in borage oil (and comes from linoleic acid). It is required to make Growth hormone and it spares the body from using glutamine.

LIPASE is secreted by the pancreas to break down dietary fat into smaller fragments. Then, further down in digestion, bile works on the fat (along with lecithin in the bile) to break it down further.

LIPID or lipids are a family of compounds that include sterols (cholesterol), phospholipids (lecithin), and triglycerides (fats and oils).

Lipid is a general term for fats. Approximately 95% of the lipids in foods and in the body are triglycerides. The two common lipids <u>in food</u> are dietary fat and dietary cholesterol. The two kinds of lipids <u>in the blood</u> are blood triglycerides and blood cholesterol.

Some lipids are essential for muscle growth and can not be made by the body. They are linoleic acid and alpha linolenic acid. Lipids are also required for the absorption of vitamins A, D. E. and K.

LIPOPROTEIN is a combination of protein and cholesterol or protein and a lipid (fat). Since lipids can not move freely through the blood, they must attach to protein for help. The two common lipoproteins are HDL and LDL which are markers for heart disease.

LIPOTROPIC FACTORS are choline and inositol. These have been shown to offset the damaging effects on the liver caused by alcohol and oral steroids.

LUTEINIZING HORMONE is a gonadotropin (released in the brain) hormone that signals the testes in the male to produce testosterone. Physical training, moderate exercise, and adequate nutrition can support the normal output of luteinizing hormone. Anabolic steroids, especially the testosterones, can cause the pituitary in the brain to stop releasing luteinizing hormone. This can lead to side effects upon the discontinued use of the steroids. These side effects include severe depression, exhaustion, irritability, malaise, and a loss of appetite. Since the body has stopped releasing the hormone, and no steroids are left in the body, maintaining muscle becomes very difficult and adding muscle is impossible as there is not enough testosterone in the body to support recovery or growth.

—M—

MA HUANG is an herb that exerts a strong effect on the nervous system. It causes the release of the stress hormone called epinephrine. This hormone causes fat cell breakdown and spares the body from relying on branched chain amino acids for fuel. The result is a loss of fat and retention of muscle. Since it has stimulatory effects, it may lead to sleeplessness and anxiety.

MAGNESIUM is a mineral that is required for protein synthesis and to release energy from carbohydrates and fat. Muscle relaxation and nerve conduction and bone formation depend on magnesium. Bodybuilders should consume up to 700 mgs a day as low magnesium levels are correlated with a decrease in strength.

MALNUTRITION is a state of poor nutrition. Those most common to suffer signs of malnutrition include pregnant women, who require more of many vitamins, minerals, calories, and protein, vegetarians who frequently lack enough iron, B-12, vitamin D, zinc, and dieters who do not eat enough food or who eat a limited variety of foods. I believe in eating a wide variety of foods and taking a quality multi vitamin/multi mineral to make sure all your nutrient requirements are met.

MANGANESE is a mineral that is required to build bones and is required for sugar metabolism in the body. It is found in whole grains and in black tea. The body needs about 2 to 4 mg a day.

MANNITOL is a sugar alcohol which can be derived from fruits or made from the sugar dextrose. It is absorbed and metabolized differently from regular sugar(s). It causes only a very small release in insulin. In pill form, it is prescribed a diuretic. It can cause a severe loss in sodium and water when taken in extremely large amounts (as in a pill).

MCT are medium chain triglycerides, a fat that is shorter in length than traditional longer chain fats like cooking oils, butter, margarine, cream, or the longer saturated fats found in meats like chicken and beef. Because they are short in length, the body can use them as fuel immediately. They also produce ketone bodies. Ketone bodies are an alternative fuel source. Every tissue in the human body (including muscle) can use ketones for fuel. Some bodybuilders on a diet use MCT to make more ketones in hopes that the body will use the ketones for fuel while dieting instead of breaking down lean body/muscle mass to be used as fuel.

MESOMORPH is a genetic body type that describes a physique that is naturally muscular and low in body fat. Almost every professional bodybuilder in the IFBB can be considered a mesomorph.

METABOLIC ACIDOSIS is a dangerous event that

occurs when the pH balance of the blood changes from normal (7.35 to 7.45). Acidosis occurs in diabetics who produce large quantities of ketone bodies which are very acidic. Extreme low calorie, no carbohydrate diets can also lead to an over production of ketone bodies that could promote acidosis. Heavy exercise can produce lactic acid which can lead to more acidic blood, but the event is not dangerous as the body can quickly adapt to smaller changes in pH. The loss of bicarbonates (which are basic in nature) can increase the acidity in the blood. Diarrhea can lead to the loss of bicarbonates. Acidosis can lead to exhaustion, low blood pressure, impaired breathing, and coma in extreme cases.

METABOLISM is the total sum of all the physical and chemical reactions in the body required to maintain life. It is the energy produced by the body. Metabolism also refers to the conversion of food to usable energy by the body.

METABOLISM OF CARBOHYDRATE. Carbohydrates are broken down from long chains (polysaccharides or oligosaccharides, or disaccharides) into glucose. All carbohydrates are enzymatically broken down into the same molecule: glucose.

MINERAL BALANCE refers to the body's natural balanced (homeostatic state) of minerals in the body. Naturally the body is made (more) of some minerals and less of others. For example, the body contains twice as much potassium than sodium and five times as much calcium than potassium. However, the American diet yields three times as much sodium than potassium which alters the mineral balance in the body. It is thought that mineral (in) balances can lead to many health problems and mineral balance is directly related to the way we eat. Bodybuilders who use diuretics severely alter the natural potassium to sodium balance by excreting sodium (from diuretic use) and increasing potassium too high with potassium supplements. The result is an un-natural potassium to sodium balance which results in muscle cramping.

MINERALS are nutrients that exist in foods and in the body. The body needs about 17 to 20 different minerals for good health. Bones, teeth, muscle, organs, muscle, blood, and nerve cells all require minerals. Minerals act as catalysts (helpers) for muscle contraction and nerve conduction (transmission) and they are needed for digestion and absorption of foods.

MONOSACCHARIDE is a term used to describe the most simple sugar: glucose.

MUIRA PUAMA is an herbal extract that can slightly increase testosterone levels in the body. It may work by improving the uptake of testosterone in the blood by the muscle tissue. This could increase muscle strength. This process also decreases the amount of testosterone that reaches the prostate gland which also has receptors for testosterone. Prostate cancer is associated with the amount of testosterone that reaches the prostate gland.

MUMIE is considered a Russian "Adaptogen". Adaptogens allow the body to recover or "adapt" to stress, such as weight training. Better recovery means more growth. There is very little scientific evidence to support the claims for mumie, but some athletes report it to be mildly effective.

MUSCLE DENSITY is a term used to describe the amount of muscle per unit of measure. Weight training increases muscle size and volume. Over time, as a bodybuilder has reached his genetic limits in size, the muscles become denser as the fibers become so thick, they "push" against neighboring fibers. This creates a super defined look as seen in the muscles of Shawn Ray.

—N—

NAD (nicotinamide adenine dinucleotide) is a coenzyme that is frequently required to <u>accept</u> hydrogen in metabolic reactions. All energy transfer in the body (for example ATP is derived from food and stored muscle glycogen can be broken down chemically to release the sugar into the blood) involves the breaking of chemical bonds. The electron transport system is a complex system where hydrogen atoms are continually stripped from nutrients during energy production. Special carriers (NAD) within the cell's mitocondria remove electrons from the hydrogen and pass them to oxygen. Oxygen then accepts <u>another</u> hydrogen to form water. All this allows energy to be produced in the body.

NATRIUM (also known as sodium) is an electrolyte mineral the body needs to absorb and use carbohydrates. It is also required for muscle contraction.

NIACIN, also known as vitamin B3 is required in carbohydrate, fat and protein metabolism. It is found in beets, turkey, chicken, fish, and seeds. It is needed to make testosterone and estrogen in both men and women and it is required by the nervous system for normal functioning. Some bodybuilders use it to increase heat production in the body. Niacin causes a small increase in body temperature which increases the metabolic rate.

NICKEL is an essential trace mineral. It is found in seafood, cereal, buckwheat, seeds, and cabbage. It helps maintain the outer structure of all cells. A deficiency in animals leads to growth retardation and poor physical performance.

NICOTINIC ACID is one of the three synthetic forms of niacin. The others are nicotinamide and niacinamide. Nicotinic acid has been shown to lower cholesterol levels in doses of 100 mg a day. Careful, this amount can cause severe dilation of blood vessels which is very uncomfortable.

NITROGEN BALANCE Nitrogen, derived from protein is usually in a balanced state. When we eat protein, the body derives nitrogen from the food. When protein is absorbed by the body and an equal amount excreted, the body is in a homeostatic or normal nitrogen balance. With an increase in protein in the diet and when the body is subjected to the stress of weight training, the body absorbs more protein, and more nitrogen is deposited in tissue. The result is a positive nitrogen balance. A positive nitrogen balance indicates the muscles are growing.

NITROGLYCERIN is a drug used to prevent angina/chest pains. It works by relaxing the smooth muscle located in the heart.

NORADRENALINE and NOREPINEPHRINE are stress hormones released by the adrenal gland in response to mental stress, fear, or exercise. They are messengers released into the blood that cause stimulation of the sympathetic nervous system. When the sympathetic nervous system is stimulated, the body increases its metabolism, it uses more fat as fuel, it breaks muscle glycogen into glucose, and it stimulates mental acuity and alertness.

NUCLEIC ACID are chemical structures that consist of a sugar called pentose, combined with one to three phosphate groups. They are important in cell metabolism. Nucleic acids form cyclic AMP and ADP and ATP.

NUTRIENT There are two classes of nutrients. The macro nutrients are needed in large quantities. They are carbohydrates, protein, fats, and water. The micro nutrients are needed in smaller quantities. They are the vitamins and minerals. The only nutrients that provide energy are the carbohydrates, protein, and fat.

NUTRITION is the scientific study of foods, what comprises them, and how they affect humans. We now know that diet can affect almost every health problem known to man, from cancer, to heart disease, to aging. Food affects the way we look and feel. A poor diet can lead to many life threatening diseases. Imagine the benefits of eating a good diet.

NUTRITION DEMAND is a term used to describe the state of the body when it is lacking a certain nutrient. A bodybuilder who has recently finished a training session may be in demand for additional protein, especially branched chain amino acids. Babies demand additional arginine and dietary fat and women demand more iron for optimal health.

—O—

OCTACOSANOL is a substance derived from wheat germ. Many athletes use this as a supplement because there have been several studies that have shown it to increase stamina and endurance by improving the body's ability to deliver oxygen to (aerobically) working muscles.

OKG is ornithine alpha ketoglutarate. This nutrient has a few unique properties. OKG is the amino acid ornithine bound to alpha ketoglutarate. It is not simply ornithine mixed together with alpha ketoglutarate.

OKG can provide fuel to the muscles to prevent muscle loss. OKG can become branched chain amino acids or glutamine if the body is low on them. It can also make KIC (ketoisocaproate) the derivative of leucine, the most important branched chain amino acid. KIC can prevent muscle break down.

Both glutamine and alpha ketoglutarate found in the OKG are good ammonia reducers. Ammonia is produced during training and from eating protein. Ammonia interferes with ATP and muscle glycogen production. The typical dose is 6 to 10 grams in the morning with food.

OKG can also become glutamine which is important as glutamine is one of the most important amino acids. It is used in large amounts during training and recovery. It is possible to deplete glutamine levels so that muscle recovery and growth becomes impossible.

OLEIC ACID is a monounsaturated fat found in both animal and vegetable sources. There are two types of fat. Saturated fat is solid at room temperature. It is the fat derived from animal sources and found in protein foods. Unsaturated fats are liquid at room temperature and is derived from vegetables. Mono unsaturated fats are a sub group of the family of fats known as unsaturated fats.

Monounsaturated fats have a positive effect on the cardiovascular system while excessive amounts of saturated fat has a negative effect.

OMEGA-3 FATTY ACID are special fats found in salmon, mackerel, anchovies, and other fattier fish. Omega-3 fatty acids can have strong effects on the body. First they work like chromium by making the receptor cite for insulin on the muscle more active. This is desirable. A sensitive receptor allows insulin (released in response to eating carbohydrate foods) to do its job: drive sugar and amino acids into the muscle for growth. Omega-3's can also increase muscle glutamine levels. Low glutamine levels as the result of overtraining or an insufficient branched chain amino acid intake will cause muscle loss. All bodybuilders should try to keep their glutamine levels high by using branched chain aminos or a wheat based protein powder, and by supplementing with 3 capsules of fish oils daily.

ORNITHINE is an amino acid that has been shown in some studies to increase the output of growth hormone in the body. Increasing growth hormone is thought to have two main benefits. Growth hormone can cause the body to hold onto more protein, creating an anabolic environment. Growth hormone also has a fat burning effect. It causes the body to shift fuel sources from burning less carbohydrates to burning more fat as fuel.

A dose of 6 to 12 grams of ornithine on an empty stomach taken before going to bed may increase grown hormone output. Eating any protein with ornithine will cancel the effects of the ornithine. Also, eating carbohydrates within three hours of taking ornithine will also cancel the effects as carbs release insulin and insulin works against growth hormone release.

OVER DIET is the term given to describe a bodybuilder who has lost muscle, instead of fat, as the result of cutting down too low on calories. To lose fat, the dieting bodybuilder should make small adjustments in his diet. Usually, fat can be lost by cutting down on the total carbohydrate intake by a small amount (10% is best). If the dieter makes too big of a reduction, fat is lost, but muscle mass is lost with it.

—P—

PABA (para amino benzoic acid) is a cousin to the B-vitamin family. It is always found with folic acid in foods like liver, yeast, wheat germ, and molasses. PABA stimulates the naturally occurring bacteria in the intestines to produce folic acid which aids in the production of pantothenic acid. PABA also is needed to make red blood cells. Red blood cells are required for muscle growth, oxygen delivery and many other processes that indirectly aid in muscle growth.

PAK (pyridoxine alpha ketoglutarate) is an easy to absorb form of vitamin B-6. It acts as a co-enzyme required to metabolize amino acids from protein and it is required to break down stored muscle glycogen to obtain glucose for the blood stream.

PANTOCRINE is a Russian supplement derived from Deer Antlers. It is supposed to increase athletic performance but probably does not work.

PANTOTHENIC ACID is also known as vitamin B-5. It is a water soluble vitamin found in higher concentrations in organ meats, brewer's yeast, egg yolks, and whole grains. It's required for the body to obtain energy from carbohydrates, fat, and protein foods. It supports the immune system and wound healing, and boosts energy levels. Most diets provide about 10 to 15 milligrams a day, enough for the hard training bodybuilder.

PAPAYA ENZYMES increase the breakdown and absorption of protein foods.

PEAKING PERIOD is the period before a contest that bodybuilders use to lose fat and hold muscle. Most peaking periods should last about 12 weeks. If you are already in good shape, you could shorten the peaking period to 8 weeks, but if you are not in good shape, you should allow for 16 weeks to slowly diet your body fat off.

PEPSIN is found in the digestive tract. It is an enzyme that initiates/begins the digestion of protein.

PEPTIDASE are found in the small intestines. Their job is to break apart dipeptides into free amino acids for absorption.

PEPTIDE BOND AMINO ACID bonds that combine two amino acids together. Two free amino acids (linked by a peptide bond) form a dipeptide amino acid.

PEROXIDE LIPID is a term given to describe a type of free radical. Muscles and tissue in the body have a fatty like outer layer. Free radicals, produced from hard training, stress, pollution, smoking, and drugs, can attach themselves to this fatty layer and poke holes in the outer surface. This leaves the cell or tissue vulnerable to a host of problems. The job of an antioxidant is to fight the free radicals that poke holes in the cell in the first place. If the antioxidants do not do their job, free radicals are produced, also known as peroxide lipids. One free radical can give way to thousands of other free radicals.

PHENYLALANINE is an essential amino acid. When taken on an empty stomach in supplemental form, phenylalanine can decrease the appetite (500 mg works well). Phenylalanine can increase the amounts of cholecystokinin (CCK) in the brain. CCK causes a decrease in the appetite.

PHOSPHATIDYLSERINE (PS) is a phospholipid. Phospholipids are a lipid (fat) similar to triglycerides but have a phosphorous containing acid in place of one of the fatty acids. Phosphatidylserine (PS) supplements are derived from soybeans. They are supposed to lower cortisol levels in the body. Cortisol destroys muscles. These supplements probably do not work as it is PS derived from cows brains (not soy beans) that have been shown to lower cortisol.

PHOSPHOROUS is a mineral needed to make bones and ATP (the ultimate and final fuel source for bodybuilding exercises). It is found in meat, milk, chicken, fish and grains. It is also needed to metabolize carbohydrates, fat and protein.

POLYPEPTIDE. Amino acids are held together by peptide bonds. A chain of protein consisting of 8 or more amino acids is considered a polypeptide. The hormones insulin and growth hormone are considered polypeptide (hormone). For example, growth hormone is a long chain of 191 amino acids and insulin is a chain of 51 amino acids.

POTASSIUM is the main mineral found inside the muscle. It is required for muscle contraction and nerve conduction. Bananas, potatoes, and meats are good sources.

Many bodybuilders use potassium supplements the last ten days before a contest. Using potassium can temporarily make a muscle feel fuller. Others simply cut their sodium. Altering the potassium to sodium ratio so the body has more potassium and less sodium can make a bodybuilder look somewhat better.

PREGNENOLONE is produced in males and females from the adrenal glands. It is a precursor to both the muscle building hormone testosterone and estrogen which can cause fat deposition. Pregnenolone also makes DHEA and androstenedione.

PROLINE is an essential amino acid (you have to get it from your food - the body can not make essential amino acids). Proline combines with the amino acid lysine and vitamin C to make collagen. Collagen is the connective tissue that binds tissues together in the body. Two of the most important collagen tissues are tendons and ligaments which are part of the joint (s).

PROSTAGLANDINS are hormone like substances that control millions of reactions in the body. They are also known as eicosnoids. They are produced naturally in the body from essential fatty acids.

PROTEIN is the body's main building material and is made up of amino acids. All of the body's tissues are made of protein including the hair, skin, muscles, blood and the brain. Protein is needed for muscle growth, and to make antibodies which fight disease and infection. Proteins also serve as a secondary fuel source for weight training. I recommend bodybuilders consume one gram of protein for each pound of lean body mass.

PROTEIN ANABOLISM results when the body is subjected to weight training. Normally the body is in neither an anabolic protein state or catabolic protein state. After training, and with the consumption of adequate protein, the body will deposit and absorb more protein (into the muscle) than it excretes. This protein anabolism leads to the increase in the size of the muscles.

PROTEIN POWDER is derived from milk and eggs which are good sources of protein due to their high BCAA content. The water content in milk and eggs is removed by either a high heat or lower heat process that absorbs all the water. The result is milk or egg powder. Low heat protein powders are best because high heat can destroy some of the amino acids in the protein.

PROTEIN SCORE is a reference to grading proteins. The accepted protein scoring system that is most accurate is Biological Value (BV). Biological value means "the amount of lean muscle weight gained by a human in relation to the amount of protein he absorbs". Milk and eggs and whey have the highest BV because they have high amounts of BCAA that build muscle and they are easier to absorb than meat and chicken. BV takes into consideration two important facts; muscle gain as opposed to weight gain (weight gain can mean fat and muscle gain!) and it takes into consideration absorption. The better the absorption, the less protein/amino acids are wasted.

PUMP-UP is a system used by competitive bodybuilders before going on stage to visually make the muscle harder or larger looking. High reps with light weight can increase blood flow the the muscles. When blood enters the muscles, they swell with blood, potassium and water. This makes the muscles look harder.

PYCNOGENOL is a name for grape seed extracts. Pycnogenol is a very strong antioxidant that has been shown in studies to be a stronger antioxidant than vitamin C.

PYRUVATE is an end by product in carbohydrate metabolism. It can be used during explosive anaerobic movements (like bodybuilding training) for fuel (as ATP) or it can be sent to the aerobic system if it is needed for fuel (again as ATP). As a supplemental form, pyruvate may encourage the body to shift fuel sources, so more fat is used for fuel. If more fat is used for fuel, a person gets leaner and spares muscle glycogen. More muscle glycogen means a better pump and more growth.

PYRUVIC ACID is another name for pyruvate.

—Q—
QUADRACEPS is the name for the 4 muscles that make up the frontal thigh.

—R—
RATIO OF FAT ENERGY is the amount of fat calories present in one's diet. Most bodybuilders will grown best on a diet that is twenty percent fat calories. A bodybuilder consuming 3000 calories daily should get approximately 20% of his calories from dietary fat. Twenty percent of 3000 calories is 600 calories.

One gram of fat yields nine calories. Therefore, 600 calories is approximately 66 grams of fat.

RELATIVE BODY FAT describes the amount of fat to muscle tissue one carries. It is a term similar to "percent body fat" where a person is trying to determine how much of their body is fat and how much is muscle.

RESERVE PROTEIN is considered the few amino acids found in the blood stream and the amino acids found in muscle tissue. When a bodybuilder trains, protein is a back up fuel source after glucose from carbohydrates. If a bodybuilder does not eat enough protein (at least 1 gram per pound of lean body weight) the body can call upon its reserves. The body will tap its own muscle, which is made of amino acids, to obtain the needed protein. This leads to a negative nitrogen balance and a loss of muscle.

RIBOFLAVIN is also known as vitamin B2, is found in meat, chicken, fish and dairy foods. It is needed to produce energy from fat and carbohydrates and is required to help make use of amino acids. Bodybuilders should consume a minimum of 50 mg a day from food or supplemental sources.

RIBONUCLEIC ACID (RNA) is a messenger that is stimulated by DNA. When a bodybuilder trains hard, eats correctly and gets adequate rest, the body releases more growth building hormones like testosterone and growth hormone. Another muscle building hormone, insulin, works better under the above conditions. Stimulation of RNA signals the muscle to increase protein synthesis.

—S—

SATURATED FATTY ACIDS are fats that are solid at room temperature. All animal fats from chicken, beef, eggs and milk is saturated. Saturated fat can lead to glucose intolerance. Glucose intolerance makes muscle cells less responsive to the body's insulin. Unresponsive muscle (to insulin) leads to a lack of muscle growth, and diabetes. Saturated fat also stores as body fat easier than other fats (unsaturated or omega-3's) and it is a factor in heart disease.

SELENIUM is another trace mineral that functions alone or with other enzymes in the body. It acts with vitamin E and the antioxidant enzyme called glutathione peroxidase to fight free radical damage in cells. Organ meats, seafood, grains and vegetables are all high in selenium.

SERINE is an unessential amino acid. Unessential means that the body can make it. Serine is required in the production of creatine the important fuel source for explosive power. Serine also combines with phospholipids to become phosphatidylserine (PS). PS has been recently shown to be an anti-catabolic by over powering the negative muscle wasting effects of cortisol. Supplement companies are making PS from vegetable sources.

SHARK CARTILAGE has been shown to exert a mild anti-tumor effect in humans. It also may fight muscle inflammation with its antioxidant properties.

SILICON is a trace mineral that is required in very small amounts to regulate metabolism. Silicon is also needed to build strong tendons, the tissue that attaches muscles to bones. Silicon is easily found in many foods, especially vegetables as silicon is absorbed by plants in the earth and passed on during human digestion.

SLOW OXIDATIVE FIBER are muscle fibers that are used during long distance and continuous activities like long distance running, and during aerobic exercise such as riding the stationary bike for 30 minutes or participating in an aerobic dance class. These fibers use primarily fat as fuel and as a result of training. The mitocondria portion of the muscle cell, where fat is used as fuel, gets bigger with consistent aerobic training. Slow oxidative fibers are extremely resistant to fatigue, unlike the fibers used in bodybuilding training which fatigue easily.

SLOW TWITCH FIBER are found in all muscle. Each muscle is made of a mix of fat twitch and slow twitch fibers. Slow twitch fibers are sometimes referred to as red fibers as they contain myoglobin, a protein that can combine with oxygen. Slow twitch fibers are resistant to fatigue and contain a much greater amount of capillaries than fast twitch fibers. Slow twitch fibers are suited for endurance activity. A person who genetically has predominantly more slow twitch fibers would not make a good bodybuilder as his body type is suited for endurance activities.

SMILAX is a plant sterol (a cousin to the steroid found in humans) that has been promoted as a testosterone increaser. Smilax will not increase testosterone levels in the body, but it could increase stamina, though to a small degree.

SODIUM LOADING is a technique used by pre-contest bodybuilders to rid the body of water located under the skin. Sodium lowers aldosterone levels - the hormone that controls sodium and water excretion. The technique I use is a high sodium diet during competition training. This is the "load". Then cut sodium, the last 2 days before the contest. Because of the high sodium intake, the body will have lowered aldosterone. When sodium is cut, aldosterone will stay low for 3 days. Therefore, the body continues to excrete sodium and water BUT there is less sodium coming in, so water is lost WITHOUT an increase in aldosterone. (Because it takes three days for aldosterone levels to change.)

SODIUM PHOSPHATE is a micronutrient and was first used by German troops in World War I as a nutritional aid to fight fatigue. One gram taken four times a day may decrease fatigue.

SPIRULINA is a plant food that is very high in vitamins. It also contains small amounts of amino acids.

STARCH is a form of carbohydrate. Bodybuilders refer to starch as "complex carbohydrates". Complex carbohydrates are found in rice, potatoes, whole grain breads, beans, and pasta.
    Nutritionists call complex carbohydrates, "polysacharides". Polysaccharides are composed of many straight and curved chains of glucose. The body breaks polysaccharides down by digesting them into "oligosaccharides" which are smaller units of glucose chains. Then the oligosaccharides are broken into "monosaccharides" or glucose.
    "Poly" means "many".
    "Oligo" means greater than two.
    "Mono" means one.
    "Saccharide" means sugar.

STEARIC ACID is an abundant fatty acid found in animals, including humans.

STEROID HORMONES include testosterone, cortisol, aldosterone DHEA, and cholesterol. Testosterone is produced by the male's testes and can increase protein synthesis in the body. Cortisol is a stress hormone and is responsible for turning body protein into fuel and breaking down liver and muscle glycogen to be used as fuel. Aldosterone regulates water levels in the body, DHEA is a weak androgen produced by both men and women, and cholesterol is needed for normal growth and the production of testosterone.

STEROL COMPLEX is found in plants. These complexes have a chemical structure that resembles steroids found in the human body.

SUBCUTANEOUS FAT is the fat found under the skin. The body also has intramuscular fat found within the muscle and internal fat that is located around the organs to act as a protector. Subcutaneous fat acts as an insulator trapping body heat in the body. It is the fat that bodybuilders try to lose to appear rippled. Average fat levels for women are 18-20% and men have average levels of 12-15%. However, bodybuilders and athletes have much less subcutaneous fat. Male bodybuilders can lower fat levels to 3 to 5% and female bodybuilders can lower their fat levels to 7 to 9% of their total weight.

SUCCINATES are compounds derived from amino acids. They can prevent the build up and accumulation of lactic acid, a by product of energy metabolism that inhibits muscle contraction. Athletes using succinates show better lactic acid clearance and greater tolerance to hard weight training sessions.

SUGAR is a general term to describe carbohydrates. Generally sugar is used to describe simple carbohydrates which are found in sweets, and fruit juices. Simple sugars break down in the body very fast while complex carbohydrates break down slower. When carbohydrates break down fast, they have a greater tendency to stimulate fat deposition.

SULFUR is present in all proteins and determines the contour of the protein. Sulphur helps specific proteins take on a special shape. Skin, hair, and nails are more rigid and contain a lot of sulfur.

SUPER COMPENSATION results when the body lacks a nutrient. If a woman's body is low in calcium or iron, the body will dramatically over or super compensate by increasing its ability to absorb both calcium and iron. The super compensation effect is seen in bodybuilders who deplete carbohydrates for three days before a show, then load up on carbs for three days. When the muscles become low in carbohydrates, they react by absorbing and storing all of the carbohydrates that are re-introduced into the body. These carbs are stored in the muscles and make them look bigger.

SUPPLEMENTS are meant to add nutrients to the diet. Pills, powders, and other types of supplements can never replace the nutrition found in foods. A person can not survive without food. Supplements should be used only to help improve the nutritional status of a person, not to replace good eating habits.

—T—

TAMOXIFEN is an anti estrogen agent used by male bodybuilders. Males who use steroids, derivatives of the male hormone testosterone, also have higher amounts of estrogen in the blood as some of the testosterone from the steroids is converted into estrogen. Estrogen can inhibit fat breakdown and promote fat deposition so the bodybuilder who uses tamoxifen hopes to lower this estrogen.

TANNING CREAMS are used by bodybuilders to temporarily color or dye the skin a darker color. Darker skin makes a bodybuilder look "harder" or more muscular as dark skin highlights muscular cuts.

TAURINE is an amino acid that has been shown to benefit the immune system. It also helps regulating blood sugar levels in a way similar to chromium. It is found in common every day protein foods.

TESTOSTERONE is the hormone produced by the testes in males that influences hair growth, facial hair growth, bone density and aids in muscle building and fat burning. Weight training increases testosterone levels in both males and females. Overtraining, training too often or too hard, can lower testosterone levels.

THIAMINE is also known as vitamin B-1. Thiamine acts as a co-enzyme in the reaction that releases energy from carbohydrates. Thiamine deficiency produces exhaustion, overtraining, loss of appetite, and tenderness in the muscles. The effects are felt by all parts of the body especially the muscles as they need the energy from carbohydrates to perform work. Male bodybuilders should get 3 milligrams daily and smaller bodybuilders (females) 2 milligrams. Liver, red meat, beans, and green vegetables are good sources.

THIOMUCASE is an injectable spreading agent used by bodybuilders. Mixing steroids and thiomucase together will cause the drug to disperse in the body faster. Many bodybuilders use it to lose water or to break down fat cells, though I feel the results are imagined or a result of continuous dieting and not the drug. Another topical cream form is supposed to cause the body to lose fat and water but I highly doubt it is effective.

THREONINE is an essential amino acid. Since it is essential, it can not be made by the body. Therefore it must be consumed every day in common protein foods. It is found in abundance in all animal foods including dairy products. It is not found in high amounts in vegetables and grins, so many strict vegetarians can become protein deficient because they can be low on one of the essential amino acids.

TIN is a trace mineral. Trace minerals are essential by the body but are found in the body in very small amounts. Not much is known of tin other than the body requires tin for growth and it is found in vegetables.

TOCOPHEROL is commonly known as vitamin E. Vitamin E can protect the outer wall of muscle cells. A lack of E or chromium, a high sugar diet, obesity, and stress can damage the outer layer of the cell which leads to stress to the cell, cell damage, and the body's inability to use glucose as fuel. This can lead to adult onset diabetes.

TRIBESTAN is a plant extract that can increase testosterone levels in males to a small degree by increasing the amount of luteinizing hormone (LH) produced in the pituitary. LH increases testosterone levels. However, when testosterone increases as a result of higher LH levels, the body eventually adapts to higher levels by producing less testosterone.

TRICARBOXYLIC ACID, KREBS CYCLE is the complex energy cycle in the body that derives fuel from both carbohydrates, fat, and protein. The end products are ATP, the chemical product used by cells for energy.

TRIGLYCERIDE is a term used to describe fat. Dietary fat is composed of three molecules of fatty acids. The THREE (3) fatty acids are considered a triglyceride. These three fatty acids (triglyceride) attach to one molecule of glycerol to form fat. Triglycerides (3 fatty acids) can be used by muscles for fuel at rest or during aerobic exercise.

TRI-METHYL-GLYSINE is a three molecule methyl donor that may improve exercise performance and decrease fatigue. This is a new supplement and has shown some promising effects in aerobic athletes and bodybuilders. It works by increasing creatine synthesis.

TRIPEPTIDE is a chain of three amino aids. When you eat protein, the body breaks the long chain of amino acids found in the food into smaller chains. Eventually, tripeptides are derived from longer chain aminos. Then dipeptides are derived from tripeptides. The dipeptides are absorbed in the small intestines.
    "tri" = 3 aminos linked together
    "di" = 2 aminos linked together

TRYPTOPHAN is an amino acid that increases levels of the brain chemical serotonin. Higher Serotonin levels seem to decrease the appetite and alter a person's mood so the "feel relaxed". Tryptophan can be used in supplemental form at 500 to 1000 mg daily to suppress the appetite. The very popular appetite suppressing drugs fenfluramine and dexfenfluramine (REDUX) work by increasing serotonin in the brain.

—U—

UNSATURATED FATTY ACIDS are found in nuts and vegetable oils that are liquid at room temperature. Unsaturated fatty acids are classified as two groups: polyunsaturated fats and monounsaturated fats.

URIC ACID is the end product of purine metabolism. Purines are found in protein foods. Under normal conditions, 90% of the uric acid is reabsorbed by the kidneys and 10% of all the uric acid is excreted in the urine. In those with gout, excessive uric acid is formed and crystals of the uric acid accumulate in the joints causing severe pain.

—V—

VALINE is one of the three branched chain amino acids. The other two are isoleucine and leucine. Valine can be used directly as fuel by anaerobically working muscles (bodybuilding type workouts). When blood sugar levels fall or when muscle glycogen levels are lower, the muscles use more BCAA as fuel.

VANADIUM is a trace mineral that can make the tissues of the body, specifically muscle mass, more sensitive to the anabolic effects of insulin. Insulin is released with carbohydrate intake and has both anabolic and anti-catabolic properties. Most bodybuilders take 2 to 3 doses of vanadium each day with carbohydrates. Each dose should yield 3 to 7 mg of vanadium. High amounts could be toxic to the body.

VEGETARIAN diets are diets that omit meats and in some cases even eggs and milk. I feel it is impossible to become the best bodybuilder possible without consistently eating meat protein. Meat protein contains all the essential 8 amino acids. The body can not make these amino acids and it requires them in the diet (every day) for growth. Vegetarians must combine different foods to try to obtain the 8 essential amino acids. It is difficult to get one gram of protein per kilo of muscle mass while eating a vegetarian diet.

VITAMINS are found in the foods we eat. They are required for normal health along with minerals and water. Carbohydrates, protein and fat are called the macronutrients while vitamins and minerals are called micronutrients. The two classes of vitamins are fat soluble and water soluble vitamins. Fat soluble are absorbed with dietary fats and water soluble can be easily absorbed directly from the intestine into the blood. Water soluble vitamins in excess pass right through the body in urine while fat soluble vitamins are stored in fat deposits. Smoking, pollution, coffee, stress, a low fiber diet, and a diet that lacks variety may either steal vitamins and minerals from the body or cause the excretion of the micronutrients.

VITAMIN A is a fat soluble vitamin found in animal tissues. It's precursor, beta carotene is found in yellow and green vegetables. Vitamin A is needed for growth, it aids in making gastric juices that enhance absorption, and it is needed for healthy skin. It also is required to make RNA, to support immunity. 5000 to 10,000 IU a day is recommended.

VITAMIN B includes 8 vitamins that function to help enzymes carry out the thousands of chemical reactions that occur in the body each day. The B-vitamins are B1 (thiamine), B2 (riboflavin), B3 (niacin), B5 (pantothenic acid), B6 (pyridoxine), B12 (cobalamin), biotin, and folic acid. Without the B-vitamins, we could not harness fuel from food. All whole grains are rich in all the B vitamins.

VITAMIN C is also known as ascorbic acid and is found in citrus fruits. It is required to form collagen - the protein required to make strong ligaments (which hold together bones to bones) and tendons (which attach muscles to bones). Vitamin C is needed to support muscle recovery, the adrenals, and to promote healing and fight inflammation. As an anti-oxidant, it fights free radicals before they can damage (muscle) tissue and it supports normal thyroid production. Most hard training bodybuilders need 1000 mg a day which is difficult to get from food along - so adding a supplement could be helpful.

VITAMIN D is found in milk and in eel, salmon, sardines, herring, and tuna. It is necessary to make strong bones and it supports the nervous system and heart. It can also be obtained through sun exposure. The sun stimulates a form of cholesterol in the skin to make vitamin D.

VITAMIN E is found in eggs, wheat germ, sweet potatoes, and meats. Vitamin E is a strong anti-oxidant. It improves glucose tolerance (makes the body use sugars better) by protecting the outer portion of muscle cells from free radicals. It aids in oxygen delivery to muscles and it expands blood vessels for improved blood flow. Bodybuilders should get at least 50 IU from their food and should supplement if needed.

VITAMIN F also known as folacin and folic acid is the vitamin that is most common to be lacking in the diet throughout the entire world. It's required to make both red and white blood cells and to make new cells for growth. Pregnant women, bodybuilders and people who drink alcohol all require more vitamin F. Anemia and tiredness are common symptoms of a deficiency. Some steroids and aspiring can interfere with its absorption. Fruits and vegetables are a good source, but it can be difficult for the bodybuilder to obtain the 400 mcg a day he needs without a supplement.

VITAMIN K is found in green vegetables, milk, and yogurt. It is required to cause the blood to clot. Aspirin can cause the excretion of vitamin K.

—W—

WATER RETENTION is associated with the build up of water beneath the skin. This can blur muscle definition. Most water retention is the result of the use of anabolic steroids which cause the body to retain the mineral sodium. Excess sodium retention attracts water. Eating a high salt diet, canned foods, and processed foods that are high in salt will contribute to water retention. Drinking more water will dilute the sodium in the body and lead to less water retention. A higher potassium intake also can inhibit excess water retention.

WATER SOLUBLE VITAMINS are the B vitamins and vitamin C. They can be absorbed directly from the intestine into the blood and do not require carriers to transport them in the blood. Any excess will be passed through the body in the urine.

"WEIGHT GAIN" POWDERS are made up of large amounts of calories - carbohydrates and protein. Carbs are needed to store muscle glycogen and to release insulin which causes protein to be deposited into recovering muscles. Protein is the building block for muscles. Muscles are made of protein. In order for muscle to grown, you need extra calories, carbs, and protein (combined with hard workouts). So, these products are very helpful. Beware, weight gain powders can also stimulate fat storage.

WHEAT GERM OIL is used by athletes as an endurance booster. Wheat germ oil contains essential fatty acids that regulate hormone production, cellular growth, muscle recovery and muscle inflammation. Most bodybuilders find better results from fish oils and borage oil supplements.

WHEY PROTEIN is derived from milk, during the cheese making process. It can be the very best source of protein for bodybuilders and health enthusiasts. Whey protein is higher in branched chain amino acids than any other protein. All bodybuilders need more BCAA. Whey protein has also been shown to be a strong stimulator of the immune systems due to its high glutamine content. A recent study in the US showed that whey protein inhibits the HIV virus in a test tube. Many bodybuilders who overtrain have impaired immune systems. Making whey protein requires that all the moisture be removed so it forms a powder. Look for a whey protein that uses a low heat drying process to eliminate moisture. Excess heat can destroy the protein! Also look for ion exchange whey protein. This process keeps all the amino acids in the product fully intact.

—Z—

ZINC is a trace mineral that is needed to make several enzymes in the body. Unlike the other major minerals:

calcium, phosphorus, sodium, potassium, magnesium, and chloride, zinc is required in smaller amounts, but the jobs is performs are very important. Without adequate levels of zinc, growth is stunted, cell division slows, immunity is weakened, the body becomes more susceptible to infections, wounds heal slower, and fatigue is common.

Zinc is found in many foods that are also high in iron. Those who tend to be deficient in iron also are deficient in zinc. Foods that are high in zinc include organ meats, lamb, oysters, shell fish, and whole grains. Zinc is often referred to as the "male" mineral. Deficiency leads to lower testosterone levels, lowered sperm count, and less mobile sperm.

The best way to obtain zinc is from foods and supplements. Zinc Picolinate is the superior supplemental form. I suggest 15 to 45 mg a day. Males and bodybuilders need more to support immunity, offset fatigue, enhance recovery, and in a man's case, keep testosterone levels optimal. Food sources include eggs, meat, oysters, milk.

NOTES

SUGGESTED READINGS

A) **Understanding Bodybuilding Nutrition and Training**
100 of the most difficult questions on bodybuilding answered by Chris Aceto.. $19.95

B) **Championship Bodybuilding**
The only guidebook available that provides the know-how and strategies to build muscle without adding body fat by Chris Aceto...$19.95

C) **The Lite Lifestyle**
150 Fat-free sugar-free recipes used by bodybuilders to acheive peak muscularity. A favorite for athletes and diabetics by Laura Creavalle..$19.95

D) **A Taste of Club Creavalle**
335 lo-fat recipes. Unbelievable variety. Reviewed 4 stars in several cooking magazines by Laura Creavalle $24.95

E) **The Health Handbook**
An easy to read - complete guide to total health. This book can be considered a summary or "cliff notes" to more complicated nutrition books by Chris Aceto................$19.95

F) **Everything You Need to Know About Fat Loss**
Fat Loss made easy by Chris Aceto............................$19.95

Please send me: Sub Total

_____ copy (s) of A $_____

_____ copy (s) of B $_____

_____ copy (s) of C $_____

_____ copy (s) of D $_____

_____ copy (s) of E $_____

_____ copy (s) of F $_____

Total Enclosed is $ _____

Make check/money order payable to:
Nutramedia, Inc., PO Box 557, Old Orchard Beach, ME 04064
www.nutramedia.com

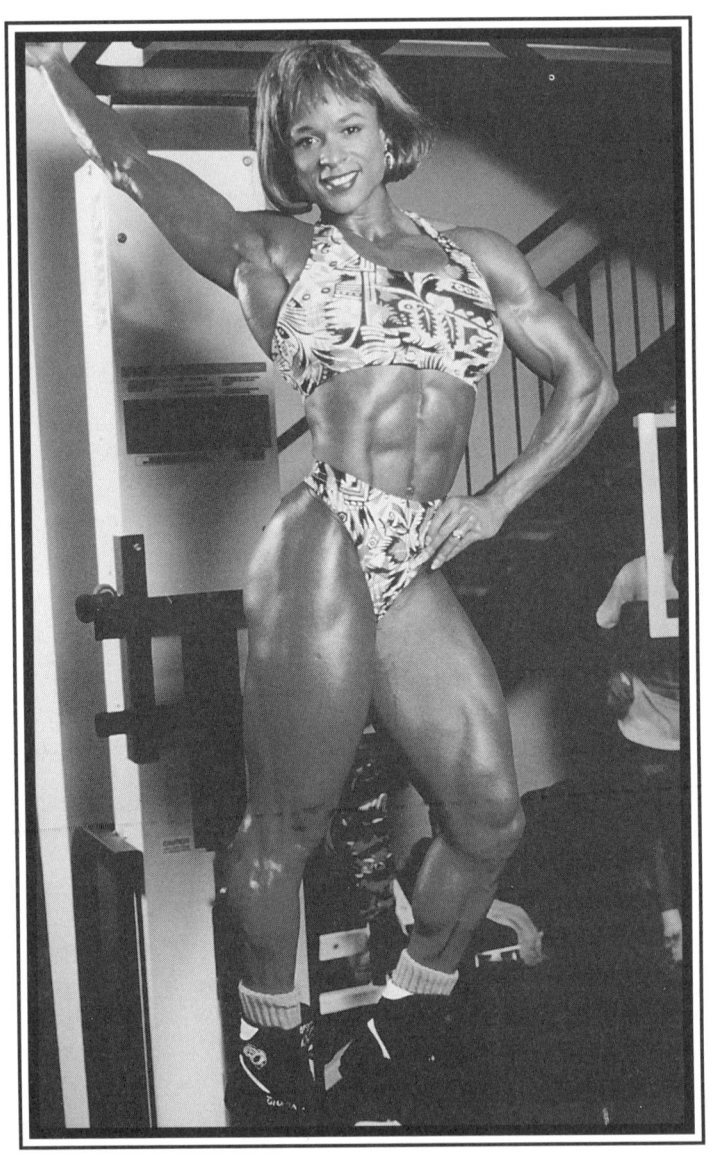

The End